Sunroofs
and
Shoeboxes

TRAIN YOURSELF TO FIND
HAPPINESS IN A COFFEE MUG,
JOY IN THE LAUGHTER OF A STRANGER,
AND **FULFILLMENT** IN THE
BEAUTY OF A SUNSET.

JAIME L. MATHEWS

Distribution by KDP Amazon and Ingram Spark (P.O.D.)
Printed in the United States of America and Canada

Title: Sunroofs and Shoeboxes
Names: Jaime L. Mathews – author
Website: www.thesweetlife.co

Paperback ISBN: 978-1-7375594-2-9
Hardcover ISBN: 978-1-7375594-1-2
E-book ISBN: 978-1-7375594-0-5

Book description: A book to help train yourself to find happiness in a coffee mug, joy in the laughter of a stranger, and mental wellness with an open Costco parking lot.

This book is dedicated to my amazing husband, Damon, my beautiful and loving children, my endlessly supportive parents, my beloved niece, and all the human and furry friends who were such a huge part of these stories. My heart is full.

Contents

Introduction

grat·i·tude (n): "The quality of being thankful; readiness to show appreciation for and to return kindness."

When was the last time you heard someone say, "I am so grateful," and actually mean it?

When was the last time you felt grateful? Not just a time where you felt lucky, but a time where your whole body and mind felt genuinely grateful and blessed all at once.

The word "grateful" is thrown around so much in our society. We send up our yogic prayer hand and bow our heads, which seems to have become the universal display of gratitude; much like the peace sign is the known signal of its meaning. But gratitude is a two-way street. It is not only the appreciation for the kindness shown to us; it is also the reciprocation of good to others. It is more than just giving thanks. It is returning that thanks so that others also have something to be thankful for. It is in these moments when we experience being grateful and in turn, our lives feel more fulfilled, healthier, and we ultimately feel happier.

So, how do you start feeling genuinely grateful?

Within these pages, you are about to read nearly a year's work of intentionally looking for health and gratitude in situations, scenarios, and during times when you might least expect it. Do you think it's possible to sit in bumper-to-bumper traffic and find something to be grateful for? Can you eat pizza and feel so good and healthy that Paleo diet followers everywhere would be utterly stumped? What about losing your pet? Can you be grateful when Fido goes missing? You can, because sometimes we have to go through a lot of gunk to be able to see the good. Each challenge or hardship offers a gift. The gift is being able to see new gold that you would have otherwise ignored. Remember, the good and the bad exist together. You cannot see one without the other.

Sunroofs and Shoeboxes shares some (actually a lot of) stories that I hope will inspire you to know, feel, and then practice seeing that gratitude, which is one of the only things we can control in our lives. When we grab hold of what our mind thinks about, we empower ourselves to experience greater health, increased happiness, and gratefulness. Are you ready?

WHAT MADE ME WRITE THE BOOK

I wrote *Sunroofs and Shoeboxes* as a way to see hope, good, and gratitude, in my own life. I was frustrated by where I was in life. I was thirty-one years old, and I always thought that by then, I would be married with children, living in a white house with a picketed fence (or something like that). Instead, I was living with a roommate, my dog, and two cats, working at my dad's business while I was also growing the hair salon I had purchased (and already disliked). Some of my friends were married, most had serious boyfriends, and I, on the other hand, had a hard time finding a date! I was so tired of being the third wheel, the fifth wheel, or even the ninth wheel at times. Not that living with roommates and animals or being single is a bad thing—it isn't! But it was not where I pictured myself in my early thirties. If I'm really honest with myself and with all of you, I was envious of my friends who had already figured out their career, and found their fella, and were playing house for real. I also knew I wanted children and the fertility clock seemed to start ticking for me around that time. I felt stuck, I felt unfulfilled, and I felt powerless to know how to get myself out of my predicament.

So as I had often done from the time I was a teenager, I started writing. Well, let's be honest, I can type way faster than I write these days, so I picked up my laptop and started typing. I decided that since I was having a hard time seeing all of the blessings I really did have in my life at that time, I would force myself to. I committed myself to writing every day for six months about the things I was grateful for. You see, I knew about the power of mindset. I had studied it constantly during my master's program in holistic health education and nutrition. I knew the power of focusing on something in order to see it. But I wasn't practicing what I preached, so I gave myself a challenge—a challenge to see good, health, and gratitude every day, even if I was having a horrible day, even if I was hung over, and even if nothing seemed to be going right in my life.

I decided to write for a hundred and seventy-seven days straight. I began writing on January 7 because beginning on January 1 seemed way too cliché for me. And most New Year's resolutions don't make it past the first month, so I wanted to set myself up for success right away. What's funny about this is that when I counted a hundred and seventy-seven days, the final day of writing landed on my only sibling's birthday. That was it! I knew I was meant to write it and I was meant to start that day. Because there's no time like the present, right?!

WHAT HAPPENED WHILE I WROTE THE BOOK

What transpired as I was writing the book was nothing short of exceptional! Opportunities started coming my way. Doors started opening while other necessary windows started closing. I was getting more and more clarity because I was focusing on seeing what was possible every day instead of what was missing. Here are a few examples:

On what I thought to be a random trip with my mom to Boulder, Colorado one weekend (laptop in hand because I did not allow myself to miss a single day and catch up later—everything had to be present day), I stumbled on a magazine. Now it's not like I found O Magazine in the bathroom and thought, "Oh cool, Oprah's favorite spring décor is here." It was Healthy Living Magazine that I was instantly gravitated to. I picked it up, read it cover to cover (and loved it!) and put it in my laptop carrying case to read again on the flight home. But it wasn't until the flight home that I discovered the advertisement for the franchising opportunity. What the what?! Me, who had a background in journalism, a background in holistic health, and loved both almost as much as coffee, could own my own magazine? It sounded too good to be true, right? Well, about eight months later, I built and launched the local edition of that magazine. And I'm telling you, I would not have been receptive to the opportunity that was staring me in the face if I hadn't been focusing on looking for what's going right in life instead of what's wrong.

Here's another example: One time during my gratitude journey, when I was eating at my favorite raw vegan restaurant, Café Gratitude, in Berkeley, California, I noticed a flyer about a three-day workshop in San Francisco that the owners were hosting. So of course, I signed up. One of the perks about not being married with children was the freedom to spend my money on whatever I wanted instead making sure the kids had plenty of school shoes. At that three-day retreat, I met some amazing people that I am still in contact with today, and I learned about a yoga retreat in Hawaii. Well, guess what? A few months after this gratitude journey ended, I was on a plane to Maui, about to embark on one of the retreats that would change my life.

WHAT HAPPENED AFTER I WROTE THE BOOK

So many things in my life began to change during and after writing the book. As you know, I found one of my business adventures with the magazine, which I sold a few years after launching. I experienced retreats that have been life changing. I have traveled to places I always wanted to see, like the Omega Institute in upstate New York.

In fact, within fifteen months of completing *Sunroofs and Shoeboxes*, I had launched and grown my magazine, I had traveled to New York City for a wellness retreat at the Omega Institute, followed by a wild and whacky girls' weekend in New York City. I hopped on a plane with my brother and then-four-year-old niece and went to Ireland to visit our godmother and travel the country, which was a trip that I will truly never forget. And the cherry on top of all of these amazing adventures was that I met my husband Damon. We met, fell in love, got married the following year, and had our twin baby girls a year after that (followed by another baby and lots of farm animals).

But let me talk about our home for just a second. One day, after Damon and I got hitched, we went for our Sunday drive. We liked to see what neighborhoods we might want to buy a house in, which schools we wanted our kids to attend—you know, married people stuff. That day, he told me he wanted to take me to one of his favorite streets. He knew I wanted a country property (even if it was a total fixer), a little slice of dirt to call our own. When he turned down the street, I was totally unimpressed. I immediately thought, "Dude, have you been listening at *all* to what I've been saying?" It was a cookie-cutter residential neighborhood, which was beautiful, but not what I was hoping and dreaming for. He said, "Just wait." As we turned the corner, the street completely changed (and we found out later that it was indeed built in two totally different time periods). The second part of the street was country as far as you could see. It was farm fencing and horses, flies and farm animals. I was hooked! We went to the very end of the street and on all the side streets, trying to look for any sign of possible home sales. Nothing. So we drove home to the house we lived in and knew we were already outgrowing.

Fast forward about a month and Damon and I drove to that street again. We now knew that we were destined to live on that country part of the street. As we turned the corner again, we saw it—"For Sale." We stopped the car, I grabbed a flyer, looked it up online and saw that it had everything we wanted in our home—the home we would raise our kids in and the home we would make all of our sweet little memories in. We went back home, and I grabbed a post-it note and wrote, "Let's get here." I posted the home flyer with that saying on it, and I looked at that thing every single day. And guess what? After several months and a little financial help from family, we got there! I still drive into my home every day and think, "Man, I am one lucky girl." Nearly nine years later and three babies, I am still living and making memories in that home and I am grateful every single day.

In addition to marriage and babies, I finally made the tough decision to close the hair salon that grew increasingly toxic for me. This was a hard one because financially, it was not a bad business. But emotionally, it was making me sick.

But the unexpected health in making those kinds of tough decisions in life is that when we choose health, it chooses us back. My husband and I decided to open a fireplace retail store and remodeling business and within five years, it has grown to a seven-figure business—a business that has enabled me to grow wings and fly, to share with all of you that the health, the joy, and the gratitude that are waiting for all of you. It might be one sunroof or one shoebox away.

The Secret of Sunroofs

As I was driving to work one day, I came across my first unexpected health tidbit. I discovered the vitality I experience from driving with my sunroof open. Okay, I didn't exactly have the chilly morning air rushing through my car, but I did have the cover pulled back to expose the sky. During warmer months, I almost always drive with my sunroof completely open, letting in fresh air and, of course, sunlight. Now that it was winter, I've kept my window to the sky closed to keep the heat in. What a waste! For those of you who have sunroofs, take this test: pay attention to the feeling you get when you have the sunroof open (at least the cover) and when it is closed. There is a distinct feeling of expansiveness when creating a little extra room and a little light in your car... and in your world. Even when the days are dreary, driving with the sunroof exposed can definitely lift your spirits.

Letting light in creates health. Sunlight provides the body with vitamin D, which is essential for all of us. Heat lamps nourish young chicks, facilitating their growth and, you guessed it, health. Light helps us see in darkness, both literally and metaphorically. If you are feeling a little dreary, as we all do at times, let some light in... even if it is just through your sunroof.

So the next time you are shopping for a new car, consider the sunroof an option worth paying for!

Music-Minded

On one Spare the Air day, in an effort to do my part for the environment, I ditched my car, strapped the running leash on my dog (I am still awaiting the day that horribly long rope trips me while running down a major thoroughfare), tuned into my favorite music mix, and away we went. The morning air was invigorating, a perfect time for some good old unexpected health revelations.

As I ran to the beat of my favorite tunes, I couldn't help but think about how healthy music can be. I stress the word *can* because as most of you know, music lyrics and artists can and have been associated with some devastatingly sad situations (take for example the song "Dust in the Wind," the song most played by people right before they commit suicide). What I mean by healthy music are those songs you sing in the car or in the shower, hum at work, run to, dance to, and maybe most importantly, those songs that elicit memories. Music creates a perfect little moment for reflection. And reflection is healthy.

How would we ever know how far we've come if we can't measure it against where we once were? Music gives us the time to reminisce about past experiences and past relationships, times of happiness and sadness, emotional growth and physical changes.

When we have these nostalgic moments, we have the choice to: a) dwell on the "good ol' days," wishing we were somewhere other than where we are right now, or b) realize that where we are today is the product of all those memories, all those experiences that we are flooded with when a song plays. Music is motivation. It can move us from a place of complacency to a place of momentum. Music can (literally!) move us out of stuck places.

So the next time you tune in to your favorite radio station, iTunes mix, or even an old-fashioned CD, remember that music will get more than your feet moving... it will get your mind moving as well.

Watch Out... and In

Once when I drove through town, I discovered some unexpected health benefits while people-watching. Let me start off by clarifying that I am not talking about making voyeurism your new hobby. But I do find that catching glimpses of others can elicit quite a sense of health and wellbeing.

Here's what unfolded: while stopped at a red light, I looked to my right and noticed three friends in their mid-twenties. I must have looked over right as one of them said the punchline of a funny joke, did something terribly amusing, or had just witnessed a comical event.

I have no idea what the topic was and it didn't matter. What I caught was one of the three laughing the most wholehearted laugh I have seen in a while. You've seen these types of laughs before, the ones that cause a chain reaction of events to occur: head tilts back, mouth opens wide, eyes squint because a face cannot possibly share both fully opened eyes and a clown-sized smile. These are the laughs that cause an almost instant grin on the face of any onlooker, and I was no exception. I couldn't help but smile and wonder, "What just gave them so much joy?" I wanted to roll down my window and invite myself into the conversation. But, in a way, I did become part of their world. I smiled because I was watching them.

It is so easy to notice the unattractiveness in people: their hot tempers, their questionable fashion sense, their size, shape, hair color, nail color... The list goes on and on. I propose that we look for the obvious qualities that create contagious positive reactions in us.

So the next time you go for a leisurely stroll, look for those who help out an elderly person. Watch for the person who picks up trash that doesn't belong to them. Notice those who let drivers *in* instead of gawking at the quick-tempered person who cuts people off. And, of course, pay attention to those who outwardly show their joyful emotions. I bet if you do, you will notice that a smile might just appear on your face. And who knows, maybe at that same moment, someone will be noticing you. Let the chain reaction of smiles begin.

Live Like You Were Living

I love Sunday mornings. You can call it a love affair. The main reason I love Sundays is the country song countdown on my favorite radio station. Now for all of my country-music-hating readers, don't stop perusing this health tidbit just yet. I promise this will not be a regurgitation of all of my favorite country song lyrics.

So one Sunday, my favorite radio station presented me with an unexpected health insight, a countdown of the top country songs of the decade. I was secretly (although not so secretly anymore) very excited to hear what the number-one song of the last ten years was going to be. I listened to the top thirteen, twelve, ten, five, four, three… and as you have already read, you'll know that I was flooded with amazing memories and experiences as each song played.

The DJ finally got to the most popular song of the last ten years and it was—drum roll please—Tim McGraw's "Live Like You Were Dying." I found it fascinating that *this* song was the number-one hit of the decade. For those of you who are not country fans, the song is a story about a son who finds out his dad has cancer and the perspective he gains when sickness and, unfortunately, death strike close to home.

You may be wondering what unexpected health has to do with Tim McGraw, country song lyrics, or a radio show. As ironic as it sounds, sickness often brings about healing, and therefore health. It may not come in the health package we think it should, but it does come. I think about the people in my life who have been sick and how inevitably healthy changes started taking place in their lives, their attitudes, and their hearts, regardless of whether their physical health changed at all.

To me, the fact that this song was the most popular song over all other country songs in the last ten years tells me that people are searching; that we as a society are trying to live life with more integrity, without so many defensive walls, and with a more forgiving, loving attitude. It shows we want to be good, loved, healthy, and happy.

The most popular song was not about drinking, cheating, calf roping, or warning mamas about having their babies grow up to be cowboys (cheesy country song joke—sorry!). It was about challenging people to live today as if yesterday never existed and tomorrow may never come.

How would we act and react if we didn't have all the protective shields we create in order to avoid being hurt and disappointed? I do not wish sickness on anyone. But I do hope that we are encouraged to live life as if we may not have another opportunity to love a little deeper, forgive those we otherwise wouldn't, and begin living the life we want to live today, and not one day later.

So the next time you listen to your favorite radio station, watch out for the unexpected health in your favorite songs—you'll be glad you did!

Re-loading Reality

Weapons, like health, create peculiar (yet very specific) images in our minds, don't you think?

I find that weapons tend to have strict descriptive guidelines: for example, weapons tend to be made of metal, wood, iron—strong elements for fending off "the enemy." Health, although perhaps a strange comparison to weapons, also takes on an image of its own: hospitals, doctors, medications, active lifestyles, eating vegetables... You get the idea. Here I go with an unexpected health tidbit: weapons are healthy and therefore, create health. Now please don't assume I am a happy member of the NRA or have a poster of Charlton Heston on my wall.

Let me explain: one day I finally saw the movie *Invictus*. For those of you who have not seen it, here's my quick Robert Ebert plug: *see it!* I give it four stars, two thumbs up, an Academy Award nomination, an MTV Viewer's Choice Award... Whatever it takes to get you to watch this movie.

Invictus exhibits what it truly means to put the past behind you and move forward. At one point in the movie, Nelson Mandela says, "Forgiveness is a powerful weapon." When I heard these words, I immediately thought about the ads I had just seen and the conversation I had just had. As

I sat and watched the pre-previews, I saw calls, advertisements to become a part of the National Guard, the Army, and I think the Marines. When I heard Mandela say that sentence, I immediately saw the pieces come together (and I now realize where most of our inspirational cards and signs originate from: the South African president himself). Without giving away the plot, weapons can be a part of health and healing, and Mandela proves this to be true. A weapon can be a wonderful addition to our belt buckle—our holster—of life.

People who voluntarily sign up to work in the armed forces are doing so (I imagine) because they love their country. They believe in a greater purpose and they are willing to fight in torrential rains, sandstorms, and other extreme conditions to prove their dedication. The weapon they enlist with is not a gun, a knife, or a grenade. It is a powerful weapon of dedication, loyalty, and love.

Weapons do not have to be items with which we kill and harm others. Discovering this unexpected insight prompted me to look up the word "weapon." Among the many killing-related definitions in *Encarta's Dictionary*, one that struck me as promising was: "something to gain advantage."

What would happen if we used weapons for healing? I wonder how my life would be different if I had love and forgiveness on my holster of coping mechanisms instead of fear and loathing. What if I chose to "gain advantage" not by trying to better myself over others but instead by creating an advantageous situation benefiting all parties involved? I'm not trying to make a political cry about the war in Afghanistan. I really have no solid ground on which to place my soapbox. But I do know that we have many battles on our own home front. If Mandela could get a nation to begin the process of reconciliation after so many years of hardship, why can't we make peace with our neighbor?

So the next time you find the idea of weapons triggering you into thoughts about the worst instincts of humanity, try to see them in a different light. I think weapons, when used in a positive context, can fight many battles, especially those battles within. Wars are not foreign to American soil. They occur on our own dirt, in our own backyards. And I highly suggest reading the poem "Invictus" by William Ernest Henley, for which this powerful movie was named.

Putting the Mind in Neutral

I am not an advocate of bulk buying. I know there are times that purchasing items in ten-pound increments is necessary, but on average, I have a hard time getting enthusiastic about going to these types of stores. Here's why: I find that these warehouses full of massive, super-sized quantities, bargains, and discounts feed our national obsession with excess.

We, as a nation, buy more than we need, more than we have room for, and more than is humanly possible to consume. So, we as a nation seem to waste more as well. But that is beside the point. I am not going to ramble on about my opinions of the Sam's Clubs, Costcos, and Walmarts of the world. In fact, I actually discovered some unexpected health one day, at a location near you!

Parking lots. Yep, there is health to be found in parking lots. As I reluctantly drove into the Costco parking lot, I turned off my car, rolled down my window enough to give the dog some fresh air, and made the long trek to the store's entrance.

Health tidbit #1 (not unexpected): These massive stores always have huge parking lots, giving us much-needed exercise while strolling from car to cashier.

Health tidbit #2 (unexpected): Parking lots are full of health elements. On that day, I felt healthy at all sorts of cement slabs. While I was strolling toward Costco, I had ample time for my ears to tune out the cars passing by and tune into the hundreds of birds that seem to perch themselves in the Costco parking lot trees. It actually never fails. Every time I have ever been to that Costco (and actually, many large parking lots that I frequent), I hear these little black birds *chirp-chirp-chirping* in the trees. And no matter what time of year, time of day, or temperature, these little feathered friends are singing away. They sing as though it is springtime, even in the middle of winter. As soon as my mind quiets enough to pay attention to my surroundings (which again, I have Costco's huge parking lot to thank), I am reminded that nature is everywhere—even in the cement jungles around us. And nature breathes health into us. Nature provides us with oxygen to live and thrive. Living organisms blossom in their surroundings, even asphalt, white-lined placeholders of vehicles.

Health tidbit #3 (unexpected): The other unexpected health tidbit I found while wandering through a parking lot was how genuine love should not be hidden, no matter who or what the receiver is. I captured a moment with an older man who was putting into his car his enormous, orange-and-white, Garfield-like cat that was almost too big for his kitty carrier. I watched, and of course smiled, at how he picked up the crate and placed it directly in front of his face, so his little buddy could see him. I heard him speaking gently to soothe his scared feline friend. This man obviously saw me: I was standing four feet away from him. But he didn't care that I was there. It didn't seem to bother him that I might have overheard a full-blown conversation he was having with a four-legged animal in a crate. Love should be this way.

Expressing love should not be reserved for the comforts of our own home. But why is it that when we grow up, it becomes easier (and less humiliating?) to smooch our pets on the corner of an intersection than our loved ones in the street? How did we get so fearful of giving and receiving love, human to human? Showing love of all kinds and to all beings creates health. I challenge us to show love with reckless abandonment of all pride, all fear, and all past hurt.

So the next time you drive into a parking lot, park a little farther away: not just for the exercise, but for the insight as well.

Caffeinated Clarity

Three easy words, one meaningful interpretation: coffee creates health.

The obvious health tidbit: coffee is full of antioxidants, acting as a disease-fighting, health-promoting substance (warning label: coffee's health benefits are measured when consuming fewer than four cups per day, more than that actually raises health concerns).

The unexpected health insight is that coffee also creates community, which creates and facilitates health. The beauty of this health insight is that even if you are not a java connoisseur (or even if you hate the stuff), you will still reap the benefits from coffee's healthiness. The nutrients are actually in the address: coffee shops.

I fell in love with coffee shops in college, deeming myself a true coffee rat (I didn't go to the gym enough to be classified as a gym rat, so there you go). I planted myself in the comfortable coffee shop seats for hours at a time, finishing homework, writing articles for the college newspaper, and eating breakfast. Coffee shops seemed to be my second home. But why didn't I just stay home, make my own coffee, and do my homework there? It definitely would have been cheaper. I know the answer. I wanted to thrive from the energy of others.

Coffee shops create that connection, bringing people from all walks of life into a cozy place built on supplying warm (or cold) caffeinated concoctions. I find that coffee shops exude the same warmth as the beverages they serve.

There are a lot of lonely people in the world: people without families, without many friends, and without the financial resources to join an adventure group, a singles group, or any other paying organization that connects people to others. And sometimes, people who have families, friends, and finances still find themselves searching for connection. Voila! The coffee shop culture began. Although I poke fun at the fact that there are (literally!) five Starbucks within a one-mile radius near me, I find it interesting that all of these manage to stay in business. As banks, phone companies, and clothing stores are merging, and car companies are closing their doors, coffee concept stores like Starbucks are flourishing, or at least staying open. I wonder if others share in my use of coffee shops: to satisfy a coffee craving and to gratify a connection craving.

I have had countless conversations while sitting at a local café. I have been challenged by strangers, inspired by those sitting on the couch across from me, and have—at times—caught up on my media gossip by a little innocent eavesdropping. In all of these instances, I was surrounded by people.

We, as a species, are not meant to be alone. We were intended to share our lives, our experiences, and our memories with others. As I write this, I think about the movie *Into the Wild*, a true story that movingly captures my written point on screen. In one scene, Alexander Supertramp (his traveler name) scribbles in his book, as he slowly and painfully faces his own fate: "Happiness is only real when shared." The brains behind Starbucks must have known this truth that Alex had to die—alone—to discover. Was the coffee culture envisioned to create the space for sharing happiness, for creating community? I'd like to think so. Because although the owners of Starbucks may be relishing their own financial success, they have also succeeded at a feat they may not even know about. They have created health by turning street-front office space into *grounds* for gathering (couldn't resist the coffee pun).

So the next time you are craving a coffee, try taking in more than the beverage: take in the community around you. There is strength in numbers. There is health in numbers as well.

Mirror, Mirror, on the Leash

Animals create health. I could start explaining why by quoting study after study about the measurable, beneficial health effects that animals have had on people (try Googling it). But if you look around, it's easy to see the health benefits constantly at work.

Pets increase their owners' physical activity. Animals are arguably the only species in our lives who love us unconditionally (sorry, parents: I think the family dog might have you beat). Furry friends provide companionship to those who lack company. However, most of all, the unexpected health insight is that animals are mirrors for us, and having the ability to see ourselves is essential for health.

My dog, Lucca, has been a mirror for me since the moment I rescued her in 2007. For anyone who has ever rescued an animal, you may have learned what I discovered: sometimes these rescue animals come with a trunk full of baggage. Packed in Lucca's luggage was separation anxiety, aggressiveness toward tall, dark-haired men with baseball hats, extreme protectiveness, and hyperactivity (she's one of the most hyper creatures I have ever laid eyes on). But I love her. With all of her wild personality quirks, she is also the most loyal, loving, and hilarious dog I have ever known.

She smiles and she talks, and her carob-chip eyebrows show expressions that are almost human.

Lucca, and any animal for that matter, is a mirror. She is a reminder that in imperfection is perfection. For some people (actually, probably for most), Lucca's individuality would be too much to handle. She could be considered high maintenance. But she fits perfectly snug into my life. Everything I used to call her baggage has actually become a blessing. Lucca's protectiveness scared away a questionable man who approached me. You better believe that guy won't be coming my way any time soon! Her separation anxiety prompted me to learn about holistic animal health (side note: I highly recommend Animal Rescue Remedy), and her hyperactivity led me to discover the wildly vast, leash-optional, open-space trails near my home, which have become my stomping grounds for inspiration. If Lucca had exhausted herself and been content with the local dog park, then I may have never discovered my outdoor playground. Lucca mirrors an essential healthy component to life: acceptance.

So the next time you find yourself baffled by the behavior of the furry friends around you, remind yourself that animals really are the same as people in some ways. Certain personality traits complement others. What one person cannot live with, another absolutely cannot live without. When we accept people and animals for who they are, we are free to live life as we are intended to. When we can close our judgmental eyes, we unshackle the constraints that we put on others and ourselves. Health is about accepting ourselves, our family, our friends, our dogs, just as they are. But I know this is not easy. In fact, I may have just lost readers. But as we are able to better accept each other, we create compassion, love, and, of course, health, in our lives. And if short- or long-term memories fail us, animals will mirror for us that when we accept others, we receive love from all over, especially from our friends at the end of the leash.

A Little Slice of Health

I discovered health in the most unexpected package. Actually, it came served on a platter, loaded with carbohydrates, processed meats, and a few scattered veggies, and is typically consumed right alongside a pitcher of beer. The pizza I am describing would not be listed in any health magazine, but health can be included as one of its many delicious toppings.

Pizza, for me, has always been centered around celebratory events: birthday parties, kids' parties, post-league sports parties, and in my most recent pizza engagement, a reunion of sorts. For nearly every important event, pizza seems to be one of those prominent features at the occasion. Pizza offers the yummy goodness we want when we celebrate happy times in life—and happiness creates health. I would argue that pizza could be classified as "happy food," not necessarily for its nutrient content, but for its quality-of-time content.

Pizza brings people together. Recently, as I sat back and watched my group of friends sitting around a table far too small for all of us, reminiscing about high school, cracking up at shared stories and, of course, eating pizza, I couldn't help but think about the irony of health. The laughter, the jokes, the funny memories and, most importantly, the people, promoted healthy living—at a pizza parlor.

In Europe, this sort of extended food gathering is not uncommon. But here in the United States, we live on the go. Our food is fast, our conversations are faster, and our chances to sit down with a friend (or better yet, a tableful of friends) are rare. But when friends meet for pizza, it is as if time, for once, doesn't really matter. In fact, I think the good old pizza pie was created in a circular shape intentionally as a reminder. A reminder that the typical reason for pizza gatherings is to celebrate with our circle of friends, to celebrate the circle of life. You get the idea.

So the next time you worry that your trip to a pizza joint is going to add a few pounds on your scale, remember that health is more than a number. Health is measurable, and sometimes it is measured not by numbers but by the quality of our days. And if spending time celebrating life means eating pizza (and possibly blowing your diet for the day), I say, make peace with the pie.

Rx: Fear for Mild Blindness

This unexpected health tidbit was revealed to me after it happened. As life sometimes reminds us, we often do not see a lesson until we are removed from the situation. For me, being overtaken by a panic attack clouded the unexpected health hidden in a heavy dose of fear. This is the kind of fear that takes over your tear ducts, causing the instantaneous floodgates to open. Let's just say I went from composed to a complete mess in approximately two minutes.

As I was walking with my dog Lucca in the open space, she stayed beside me, as she always did, without a leash. Then something spooked her and she turned around and ran, full Lucca-speed, toward I don't know where.

Let me start by saying that Lucca is fast—greyhound fast! And, as I already mentioned about her baggage, she would never, ever, go to anyone if I wasn't around. To top it off, the streets near the open space are busy. This combination of her personality traits and the surroundings made this dog owner a little scared to say the least. In a split second, she was nowhere to be found.

After I went sobbing to my parents' house, hoping she had run there, and then back to my house to fetch my cell phone, my roommate and I sped off down the street to find her. After about an hour from separation to searching down streets, I saw my little, black, carob-chip-eyebrowed, heavily panting dog running down the *middle* of the street. Way to make a statement, Lucca!

But the unexpected health is not another "animal as mirror" story. It really is about fear. Here is why fear is healthy: what I didn't mention in my long, dog-gone-missing story was that as soon as I showed panic, anxiety and fear, people immediately came to my aid (except for the poor kid I yelled at when he rudely shunned my question: "Have you seen a black dog running around here?" Sorry for the name-calling, buddy). Approximately one minute into me telling my lost dog story, I had four people I'd never met offer to drive around the neighborhood and look for her. Total strangers! And as soon as I told my dad and roommate what happened, they dropped what they were doing and headed toward their cars before I could even windshield-wipe away the tears that had built up on my sunglasses.

When we show fear, we show vulnerability. And being vulnerable is a healthy place to be. When we are not at our strongest, we allow others to help. This creates health for both the receiver and giver. When we reveal paralyzing fear, we give others the opportunity to show us how much we are loved and cared for. Even complete strangers want us to be happy. People feel good when they are able to help others. No matter how much we gripe and complain about being over-extended in life, we humans have an innate desire, a need, to help friends (or strangers) when they could use a hand. We truly are never too busy to help—and today was no exception.

Not all fearful situations turn out as lucky as mine did, I know. But I find it remarkable that when we are at our weakest, and possibly overtaken with fear, we can still feel healthy. We can even help others feel healthy, too.

So the next time you get yelled at by some wild-eyed, crazy lady uttering strange things out of a car window, don't take it personally. Maybe she just lost her dog.

Mug Shots of Meaning

I suspect that most people, like me, have at least one kitchen cabinet full of mismatched glasses, cups, and mugs. If so, you understand the frustration when trying to unload the dishwasher. The art of getting all that glassware to fit on the shelf is like trying to match the first few pieces of a puzzle (nearly impossible). But the unexpected health insight of the day is not about the healing properties of clearing out the clutter in your life, although the health benefits of spring cleaning are exponential. As crazy as it sounds, health can be found in coffee mugs.

The substances that go *into* coffee mugs have all sorts of known health benefits. We have already covered coffee. And teas of all varieties are full of aiding properties: antioxidants, stomach soothers, calming nighttime remedies, digestive aids. But what I'm talking about is the health benefit from what is printed *on* the coffee mugs.

As I spent the day in my office working at my various projects, I had many moments when I found myself daydreaming. This happens often… I'd like to say it is a writer trait but I'm afraid it is just a poor attention span.

In one of my lost-in-la-la-land moments, I caught a glimpse of my coffee mug. I looked at it and then immediately went to my kitchen, tore open my cabinet, and began poring over the words on each cup. As if that wasn't enough, I then opened the dishwasher, pulled out the rest, and read those, too.

What I realized is that I intentionally buy and use specific mugs based on how I feel or want to feel. And because of that, I have jammed my coffee cup shelf with meaningful and inspirational mugs. A few of my favorites: "God danced the day you were born," "Just when the caterpillar thought the world was over, it became a butterfly," and, "Not tonight dear, I've got a deadline." As you can see, the first is a reminder of my existence (given to me by none other than my mom), the second reminds me that when I'm feeling stuck in a cocoon, it is only temporary, and the third is a reminder of my gift of writing whenever I doubt my skills (this was an award I won for an article I wrote for my college newspaper).

It is easy to forget how special we are. Life can dish out some pretty tough times that make us question who we are and what we can possibly contribute to this world. When this happens, it is essential to remind ourselves, daily, of our uniqueness. Because our uniqueness and our gifts allow us to experience health ourselves as well as facilitate health in others.

When we are living to our fullest potential, we are experiencing health. And coffee mugs, with their eclectic words, art, and expressions, create perfect little hand-held reminders of how great we really are.

So the next time you do some kitchen cleaning, remember to keep those meaningful mugs. Not only will your body be renewed by a mug's liquid love, your spirit will be rejuvenated by its inspiration. And when you reach for your next holder of beverages, pay attention to the mug you choose. It may contain a visual inspiration you need to read today.

Weekly Wisdom

Mondays get a bad rap. This poor, innocent day—no different from any other day ending with Y—is tainted with sad phrases like "the Monday morning blues." Even songs were created to mourn this seemingly dreadful day ("Manic Monday," "Monday Monday," "Come Monday"). What is it that the Bangles, the Mamas and the Papas, and Jimmy Buffet thought was so terrible about starting the week? But (cue music) while Monday begins the work week, it also kick-starts any week by penciling in a little unexpected health.

Monday is the depressing reminder that the weekend is over, right? The alarm clock goes off and we roll over, thinking that only nocturnal creatures should be awake at this hour. We grudgingly make our way to the bathroom to begin our morning routine. The bathroom light is too bright for our sleepy eyes, the bathroom floor is freezing, the towel is still in the dryer from yesterday's wash (but you don't realize that until you've already showered)! Oh, to be able to wake up and have it be Sunday. How many times have you thought that?

But Monday provides us with a clean slate, and having the opportunity to start fresh is healthy. From diets and fitness programs to new jobs and new perspectives, Monday is the foundation for transformation: for bettering ourselves, our lives, and our circumstances. When we want to challenge ourselves, we start on Mondays, not Sundays. So, why do we mourn the day that gives us the green light to go ahead with our lives? As unexpected as it sounds, our health is actually enhanced because of Mondays!

Weekends are necessary. They are intended for relaxation, rest, and time to catch up with loved ones and friends. But weekdays are necessary too. They create much-needed outlines for our lives. Weekdays provide schedules to keep us focused on the goals and aspirations we want to accomplish.

So the next time Monday morning rolls around, try putting on a different life lens: when you turn off your alarm clock, sit in bed for just a moment and remember how healthy Mondays are. And if you ever run into a songwriter, suggest they start writing songs about Tuesdays.

Physical Health

Have you ever had a day where you couldn't spot anything good? Where you couldn't find any health benefit to any action you were doing? Or where there was nothing happy going on in your world? We have all had one of those.

I had one of those days a long time ago, where it seemed painfully difficult to find unexpected health. In fact, I had a hard time spotting any health. I could have been sipping a smoothie out of a coconut while doing yoga on the beach and I still would have missed the health insights. Instead, here's what my seemingly blind-to-health eyes focused on: buckets of rain, dark, dreary clouds, thunder that scared ten years off my life, incredibly expensive espresso machines that break, electrical outlets at the salon that never seem to work. And why am I carrying around this sopping wet umbrella that is actually dripping water on me, indoors? That is the kind of day I was having. But as my eyes re-focused (at nearly 10 p.m.), I discovered it: the health that is found, unexpectedly, from physical contact.

Now you might be thinking that there is nothing unexpected about the health benefits of physical contact. You might even be able to pull up the *Journal of the American Medical Association* archives and find a few studies. But what is unexpectedly healthy about physical contact is that you are forced, physically, to remove yourself from your own world. And being aware of those around us is healthy.

As I lay down to write my daily insight, I stared at my computer screen. For once, I had nothing to say, nothing to write about, and definitely nothing healthy to share. After gazing at a blank screen for many minutes, I felt my left arm weighed down, too heavy to keep propped up on my laptop, which meant I could not type. I felt my Siamese cat Riley nestled up against me, taking over nearly my entire arm. These sorts of shenanigans do not help a girl write! My first reaction was to get a little perturbed. But I couldn't help but smile, forget about my problems of the day, and just pet him. He made it very clear that there was something more important to pay attention to than my electrical outlet problems.

Life is full of headaches. We all have them. But what if we shifted our focus? What if we remedied some of life's aches and pains not by an over-the-counter pill but by physical contact? Studies have shown that physical contact is essential for children's growth and development. Their health is directly dependent on others. But so is adult health. Deep down, we are all just kids inside, disguised as adults. Our basic survival needs are still the same as when we were young.

So the next time you are having one of those days when the clouds seem to follow you, remember that, instead of pushing others away, you should draw them closer. You might be amazed at how good a little physical contact can make you feel.

Wintry Wisdom

Winter weather can be bothersome. After taking the time to get ready, we walk outside only to have the hair that took us ten minutes to perfect either blown into a perfect bird's nest or rained on to look like a dog after a bath.

If you have short hair, you may not have this problem, but I'm sure everyone can relate to the annoyance of having to do life in extreme weather conditions. If I were sitting in my house drinking hot cocoa and watching the wind blow or the rain fall, I wouldn't mind it at all. But ask me to run to the grocery store in those conditions and I think I'd opt for a winter fast.

The health found in sunny conditions is well-documented: vitamin D and increased serotonin levels being outdoors. I mean who doesn't love a warm sunny beach day?

We tend to forget the health benefits of a cold rainy day. You are probably reading this right now and can't even think of any. Why? Probably because you are remembering your case of Seasonal Affective Disorder (SAD) during the last cold and rainy season. SAD is a health issue that many people face during winter months—an actual medical condition. You don't find much medical research on the health benefits of winter or its weather. But wintry weather is actually full of unexpected health. You just have to see it to believe it.

Weather (in particular, winter weather) creates a perfect visual and tactile depiction of health, and being able to see and feel health at work is, in itself, healthy. Consider these windy metaphors: "the winds of change," "throwing caution to the wind"… You can feel wind blowing through your hair, which can be a reminder to change your perspective.

Wind can nudge us (or almost knock us over) with its power and presence, and so can change. Change, like wind, can be scary. It can rattle us, just as wind shakes up the trees. Wind, like change, leaves an imprint. After a howling wind, the scenery is never the same. Change changes us, and that is healthy. Because as we get rattled, shaken up, and swirled about in life, we gain insight. We learn. We eventually walk around the pothole instead of repeatedly stepping in it.

So the next time you grumble about the scenery outside, remember that this wintry weather is a visual into our internal scenery. We cannot live without the winter weather, and we cannot thrive without some vigorous change.

The Wait Gain

I would not classify myself as a patient woman. If my family and friends spouted out my greatest qualities, patience would probably not be on the top of their list. I do not like to wait for people, for surprises, or for traffic lights. I am annoyingly punctual because I don't want people to wait for me (but only because I dislike waiting for others).

But I have discovered the unexpected health in lateness. I preface my unexpected health explanation with this disclaimer: I am not advocating lateness. There are many unhealthy consequences of being late: stress hormones, high blood pressure, irritability, irrational driving—you get the picture. But there is abundant health in waiting. Waiting forces you to creatively pass the time and this practice is healthy.

True to form, I arrived five minutes early to a health and wellness presentation I was speaking at one night. I had to stand outside and wait for the previous meeting to end so I could go in and set up. As I stood outside the meeting room, I started looking around. What could I go look at to pass the time? My cell phone was off so I couldn't check my email, text someone, or do anything else that made me appear important and technologically savvy. I waited and

I waited. The meeting was running late, so there I stood, waiting (and sighing, I'm sure). But the longer I stood, in the dark, the more I listened. And eventually I heard the music. As I pinpointed where the music was coming from, I looked over and saw a church. In the darkness of that rainy night, I saw a whole wall of stained-glass windows, lit up by the light shining on whoever was practicing the piano. That's all I could see. Red, yellow, green, blue, orange, and purple rectangular slits of light radiating against the black that surrounded me. While I had scurried in, making sure I was punctual, I completely missed the light show. And had the meeting finished on time, I would have missed it again. But for once I was thankful for lateness. Someone else's lateness gave me a gift of light.

We are a society of busy bees. We schedule our time to the minute. We schedule time to make our schedules. But life doesn't always happen according to plan, and health doesn't either. Sometimes, some of the most amazing, most profound events and experiences happen during the in-between times, those times before or after the big events we think are going to change our lives.

So the next time you are caught in the waiting game, remember the health, the *aha* moments, and the "wait gains" that often unfold during the down times.

A Little Dose of Losing

I am not a sore loser. I just find any sport much more fun when my team wins. I don't throw my tennis racket against the fence or kick volleyballs around the court after a lost match, but let's face it, who likes losing? However, tonight, after volleyball games both lost and won, I found the hard-hitting unexpected health in losing.

To lose something, whether it's a game, your car keys, or even feel like you're losing your mind at times means to have something taken away. But what if we thought of losing differently? What if what we had taken away was something we didn't need anymore? I'm not talking about losing a loved one or any sort of tragic event. I would never make light of something so incredibly sad. What I mean by losing are those less heavy-hearted events that throw us into unnecessary emotional turmoil. As we are able to keep a level head, we are practicing health.

Let's go back to my sportsmanship, which is how I came to discover the unexpected health insight. One night I went to open-gym volleyball. I love volleyball! And I have been playing for a very long time, so as you can imagine, I know what it feels like to be on a winning team, and I know what it feels like to be the losers.

My team that night had an interesting dynamic. We couldn't quite connect. We somehow managed to win a decent number of games, but I never really felt like a winner. In fact, what I noticed was that the team that lost most games had the strongest connection as a unit. This made me think about winning and losing. Having something taken away from us, losing, can be really healing. When we feel like we have lost control, lost our way, lost our sense of purpose, we are given an opportunity. When we lose, we can either think the worst and believe that we must have the word "loser" stamped on our forehead, or we meet the challenge to let go of what was taken away and prepare ourselves for what will be given to us. What a great challenge, in sports and in life!

So the next time you lose something, before the irritation kicks in, think about what unexpected health you might gain from your loss... Maybe losing isn't so bad after all.

Table for One

One night, I conducted an experiment. And as expected, I came away with an unexpected health insight: the health we experience from being alone. Let me first differentiate between being alone and being lonely. Being alone is literally being by yourself, but there are no emotional connections involved. Being lonely, on the other hand, implies a sadness from being without another. My unexpected health came from being alone.

Back to my experiment. I met my good friend as we were beginning our girls' weekend to South Lake Tahoe, but before we headed up the mountain, she had a client dinner she had to go to. So, we went down to the hotel bar to wait for her client. Her client came about fifteen minutes later and they headed off to the restaurant. The plan was for me to meet up with the dinner party afterward, so I had brought my laptop to the hotel room so I could go up and write while my friend was eating. Well, after they left, I decided to stay at the bar and just people watch. But I also had an ulterior motive. I wanted to see how long I could just hang out at a bar by myself on a Saturday night without using my phone (or alcohol) as a crutch.

So there I sat. I even stayed at a table right near the

entrance, so there was no hiding or lurking in the corner of the bar for me. I could have easily bellied up to the bar, reenacting a *Cheers* episode, but I didn't. I also made sure to keep my phone in my purse and only allowed myself to have my small notepad out to take down any thoughts I had. Well, my pen nearly ran out of ink from all the insight I gained from being alone. But the most poignant unexpected health I discovered was that being alone makes you appreciate others, and being grateful for people in our lives is healthy. I have always enjoyed time to myself. But what I found is that I enjoy time to myself because I know that I will soon be surrounded by friends and loved ones. Sitting in a room full of conversations, interactions, laughs, and stories shared between friends made me appreciate that although I was sitting alone for a few hours, my aloneness had a time limit. I knew that eventually, I would reconnect.

We all need times of being alone and times of being together. I once heard this fantastic little nugget of wisdom: "You have to go in to go out." This is an important practice. When we are alone, we gain perspective. We have the opportunity to contemplate our lives, our decisions, our goals. These times of being alone prepare us to live the healthiest life when we are out in the world.

So the next time you are given the opportunity to be by yourself, take it! Put away your cell phone, your laptop, and your work and just be. It is a little awkward. It feels a little uneasy, I'll be honest. But the insight (the health) you experience from the journey alone equips you to better connect to the next person about to enter your life… or sit at your table.

Traveling Toward Health

After an amazing weekend of sleeping in two different hotels, driving six hours or so, skiing, gambling, and eating at a multitude of restaurants, I was happy to throw my stuff on my bed and be home. As I unpacked my things, I thought about how healthy it feels to be at home. You cook what you want, you sleep in your bed, and your clothes fit nicely in your closest instead of stuffed in a bag. But when I thought about all of the weekend's meaningful conversations, the laughs, and the memories, I found the unexpected health at home... But not the home your mail is delivered to. Being at home with who you are no matter where you physically land is healthy.

Home is typically associated with a nurturing warmth, a place of reprieve and rejuvenation. But not everyone has a house. There are many people who have no place to call their own. There are many whose home is full of chaos and sadness. But home can mean so much more than a roof over your head. Although I was hours from the place I hang my hat, I felt right at home because my surroundings and company helped create a homey environment and because of that, I felt healthy. I didn't eat my daily dose of vegetables, and I didn't get eight hours of sleep each night, but I found essential nutrients in my surroundings. Health is abundant when we are able to surround ourselves with those people and places that promote our growth and expansion.

I am eternally grateful that I have a roof over my head, and that I am so welcomed at my family's house that I still have a key. But even when I am far from both, I discovered that I can metaphorically pack my home with me wherever I go.

So the next time you are away, far from your loved ones and a long way from where you live, remember to pack your bags with those essential elements that create home and ultimately, health. When you surround yourself with healthy surroundings and people, home can be experienced in any zip code.

Keep Going and Going and Going for Health

Nike gear shouts from the shirt, "Just Do It." Chase Bank advises, "Chase What Matters." Safeway provides "Ingredients for Life." And evidently, we're all in "Good Hands" with Allstate.

Corporations have been criticized for years: the corruption, money-making agendas and oftentimes unacceptable working conditions have put big-money organizations on the radar of countless consumers, and rightfully so! But discovering unexpected health in the big, bad world of corporations like MasterCard is "Priceless."

I am a sucker for slogans. I remember catchy songs, I cry at commercials (some of those MasterCard commercials are actually pretty priceless!), and I love nothing more than to hear a good slogan. But as I was listening to the radio today, I realized that although corporations may be riddled with corruption, greed, and monopolizing tactics, their slogans are unexpectedly… healthy.

I have crawled up on my soapbox more times than I would like to count, pointing my finger at how large corporations are taking over the world, putting small, mom-and-pop places out of business, building on every available square inch of the universe, and creating mass consumerism (remember my Costco rant?). These may all be true. In fact, I am in no way saying that corporations are healthy. But just like the birds in the Costco parking lot, it is possible to discover and facilitate health in the most unlikely of places... And the health in corporate slogans is no exception.

If you pay attention to common themes in corporate slogans, you will notice that they offer incredibly healthy suggestions. Consider these major campaigns: "Just Do It" (Nike), "Chase What Matters" (Chase Bank), "Ingredients for Life" (Safeway), "Moving Forward" (Toyota), "Thrive" (Kaiser Permanente), "Moving at the Speed of Life" (Shell Oil), "Play. Laugh. Grow." (Fisher-Price). All of these slogans encourage health. These corporations create snappy little sayings that we remember. The key is to remember what the slogan says instead of focusing on the corporation the slogan is representing.

We all need some healthy reminders sometimes. We would benefit from just doing it. We need to remind ourselves to play, to laugh, and to continue growing. And we could all benefit from chasing, or focusing on, what matters in life. It is easy to focus on the negatives. Our time can so easily be spent berating the corporations, the people, and the experiences that create dis-ease in our life. But what would happen if we actually took the advice of these corporations? How would our health change if we started moving at the speed of life instead of being stopped by the speed of disarray? Health is ever evolving.

So the next time you hear a catchy song, a witty saying, or watch a memorable commercial, remember what I've said... Health is embedded in slogans. Can You Hear Me Now? Good.

Reading Between the Lines

When I was young, you couldn't pay me to read. Literally, my parents tried bribing us with the whole penny-per-page trick and even that didn't work! Of course, my brother, being the entrepreneur he has always been, poured through books, inevitably cashing in on the reading proposition. I, on the other hand, could not be bothered with reading, no matter how much money was involved. I had much "better" things to do than sit around with my nose in a paperback. But the activities that once brought us joy and ultimately, health, do not necessarily grow with us. Reading has become a healthy and gratifying pastime for me... And along the way, I have flipped through pages full of unexpected health.

Reading is healthy for all sorts of reasons: it elicits relaxation, occupies our minds, tunes out our chaotic world, befriends lonely souls with stories of grandiose adventures. But the unexpected health insight is that reading causes sharing. The words formulated to create a good story give us permission to share, and sharing is not only healthy, it is essential.

A while back, my good friend sent me an article about a hundred-year-old woman who received her bachelor's degree... Three weeks after turning a century old and one day before she died in her bed. After I read the article, I was inspired. But the unexpected health insight I gained was the reading itself. Reading causes a chain reaction. You read something, you likely or hopefully pass it on. When my friends and I read a good book, instead of collecting dust on a shelf, we pass it around. Reading promotes the exchange of knowledge, lessons, and truths about life, love, and all other experiences in our lives.

We don't have to be published writers to inspire others with our story. And we don't have to be speed readers to retain the wisdom of words. Sometimes health comes in a two-sentence email from a friend. Other times health is experienced through a story we read in the newspaper. But most times, health is enhanced by reading.

So the next time you open an email, check your text message, or read a story, remember to turn on the reading light to health. And when you read something remarkable, pass it on.

Take the Challenge

We all have challenges in our life. We get a challenging task at work. We challenge ourselves to train for a marathon. We have challenging kids in our classroom. We are confronted with a challenging person.

Challenges are everywhere. A challenge pushes us, providing us with a constant reminder that life is not always a frolic through the tulip fields. And because of that, I find that being challenged provides us with not only a story to tell at the dinner table, it presents some unexpected health in our lives.

Challenges give us circulation, and being stirred up in life is healthy. Have you ever watched a fountain that is not working properly? When the fountain pump is not circulating water sufficiently, the end result is an algae-filled pool of water set in a three-tiered pile of cement. What was once a vision of relaxation and soothing sounds can quickly become an oversized science experiment on living organisms. All because the water lacks circulation.

Our bodies are over seventy percent water, so it is no surprise that we find health in something that circulates. Now, I'm not necessarily talking literally about circulation in our bodies. I am not advising you to go sign up for a round of colonics (although they seem to have some health benefits as well). What I mean by circulation is the movement that happens when we are challenged.

When we are presented with difficulty, we have no other option but to shift. We shift our physical position. We shift our eyes. We shift our perspective. Challenges remove us (sometimes gently, sometimes abruptly) from our cozy little comfort zones. And when we get shaken out of our tree, when we are challenged, we can either hit the ground or hit the ground running toward a solution. We facilitate, promote, and encourage health when we take action in our life. We reap amazingly healthy rewards not after we continue to do life the same, but when we rise to the occasion of a challenge.

So the next time you are faced with a difficult decision, a frustrating person, or a trying task, remember that a little bit of health could be circulating through.

Internet Introspection

I have a love/hate relationship with the internet. I love that I can access just about anything anytime, anywhere. I hate that the internet has created scary things like online exploitation. The creation of the world wide web is a mixed bag of treats and treacheries. But spun into the amazing opportunities and the horrible detriments that make up the internet, you can load up your toolbar with unexpected health.

The internet is literally a web of connection, and being in the know of your surroundings is healthy. Let me be more specific. Remember MySpace? I thought it was a sleazy attempt at connecting friends and those who wanted to be your friend (or more!). I admit that I had an account, but I never thought much of it and was never an active user. So, imagine my reaction when this Facebook thing came out. Another excuse for peeping toms to peruse my personal pictures, information, and life, right? Not at all.

Facebook (and other online resources for webbing people together) is this amazingly healthy presence on the internet. Being a part of the Facebook world shows me the amazing humanity I am surrounded by: strangers helping strangers, amazing organizations providing for those in need, even police officers helping a homeless man shave his face for an interview. Is all of Facebook's content like this? Of course not. But I choose to stop my scrolling finger on these types of posts.

So the next time you feel like ranting about the ills of the internet (and like I said, there are lots of things to rant about!), remember the incredible opportunities it creates for us humans. We are all in some way humanitarians. We have to be. The word does not have the same meaning without us humans in it. We all get that heart tug when something, someone, or some event touches us in a way that makes us fight back tears. We're meant to. That's what makes us human. And that's what makes us healthy. Even if we are busy doing life, humanity shows through, even through the internet. If we create our world to be too busy to interact, to reveal our humanity and see the humanity in others, life has a funny way of opening up a window of opportunity... And sometimes, it's a webpage.

Painting My Self-Portrait

I am borderline OCD. No clever acronym... I am actually referring to the medical term that actors like Jack Nicholson perfectly portrayed in *As Good As It Gets*. I have a little bit of Obsessive Compulsive Disorder.

Having OCD means I have to make my bed every single day before I can leave the house. I wipe down my bathroom sink so I never have water spots on my faucet. My dresser drawers, closet doors and kitchen cabinets are always closed. And yes, I organize my food so that all the labels face the same way. For all of you fellow OCDers, I know you can appreciate what I just described.

One day, my OCD kicked into high gear; but as I one-track-minded my way through the day, I discovered some unexpected health in painting.

I got the creativity itch to paint my office. Now most people who get an idea like this may put it off for another few weeks or months. They would most likely go to the local paint store and bring home color swatches to tape on their wall to ensure they pick the perfect color. Not me! I had the idea and within an hour, I was at the paint store getting my colors mixed. OCD? Possibly. But painting has lots of therapeutic purposes. A relaxing way to pass the time, it creates newness in an otherwise old room, and signifies a fresh start.

The unexpected health I found while painting came from the color. Color allows you to paint your environment whatever color you want, whatever color resembles you, and being able to express yourself is healthy. The color I chose was called Kentucky Bluegrass, so as you can imagine, it's a *big* color! My walls make a statement. And that is exactly what I wanted. I have read enough about feng shui to know that your office, your space to create, dream big, and make a statement in this world with your business, is supposed to be filled with power colors. Colors that elicit a sense of boldness. Well, Kentucky Bluegrass (turquoise, but brighter and greener) was my power color. And as I rolled the color on my wall, I couldn't help but smile at its vibrancy.

Painting and paint colors are full of healing and health. When you put a fresh coat of paint on a wall, you get to express yourself on a large canvas. You can create the experience you want to have in a room. Obviously, Kentucky Bluegrass would not be appropriate in my bedroom because I don't want that personality trait (you know, the borderline OCD) to be active in my sleeping haven. But in my office, where I want to write, express and be bold in this world, that's the perfect place for a little *big* in my life.

So the next time you go shopping for a wall color makeover, consider the room you are painting. Be bold if the surrounding applies, be calm if you want to unwind, and create warmth in the rooms for sharing life together. Remember, the nearly endless color swatches at the paint store are there for a reason. We all have colors that represent who we are and how we feel. Sometimes we need permission to unlock ourselves, and paint gives us the stamp (actually, swatch) of approval.

Heart Healthy

February is Heart Healthy month. Not only is it the month when chocolate heart boxes, heart-shaped balloons, and candy grams overflow the grocery stores, it is also the month to promote health for our hearts. This alone is healthy. We have a month designated to eat foods that promote a healthy heart (healthy fats like avocados, raw nuts and seeds, vegetables of course, fish oils, and a little hawthorn berry extract). We have twenty-eight or twenty-nine days dedicated to exercising our heart with cardiovascular workouts and of course, February is the traditional month for cupid to launch his love arrow toward all the couples in the world. And one February, I discovered some unexpected health insight... in love.

Most of us can relate to the feeling of being in love. We feel a greater sense of happiness, excitement. You could even say that our hearts feel bigger and beat stronger when we are in love. But today, I learned that love is not a feeling, it's a choice. And having choices in our lives is healthy.

We can have feelings of gratitude, appreciation, and dedication toward others. These feelings, along with a slew more, allow us to love another. It is the combination of these warm and fuzzy attributes that help us pick our partners, who we then choose to love. The most essential need we all have to give and receive is love, but it does not necessarily come in a heart-shaped box with See's chocolates inside. To choose love, we choose to love those who may not give us the warm and fuzzies. In fact, if we choose to love, we are making a choice to love those who may downright annoy us. But a human's greatest gift, the healthiest practice we have in our gym bag of life, is to love. It is good for our minds, good for our bodies, and definitely good for our hearts.

So the next time February comes and goes, remember that the most health-promoting activity you can do requires no gym membership, no running shoes, and no hawthorn berry extract (although these are all very heart-healthy too). When you see the heart-shaped overhaul, consider this a reminder to practice the most essential human gift we have: to love.

Getting in Shape

I am going to start this with a little bit of tooting my own horn. I would like to refer back to the health benefits of Mondays. Yes, the measly start of the work week, the day that people dread, write songs about and downright loathe at times. Well on another random Monday, I discovered all kinds of unexpected health tidbits. I am not proposing that Monday be yet another piece of unexpected health… Instead, health is found abundantly in circles.

The shape of a circle is a meaningful representation of all sorts of health: it signifies an unending of sorts. Circles represent togetherness. There are no edges in circles, creating a cohesive pattern of movement, but tonight, circles meant commitment. Circles remind us of where we've been and where we're going, and coming full circle is healthy. It's not to say that we ever arrive, but when we can stand in the exact same place and be completely different, there is substantial health in that.

One of the most treasured people in my world got engaged on that night. Talk about circles! A circular band of diamonds rested on her dainty little ring finger. We all sat together (in a near circle) celebrating the newest chapter she was about to start in her life. But as I thought a little more, health kept circling around my mind. We all come to a time when we can sit back as almost an outsider to ourselves and see how our life has come full circle. That night, I saw the full circle movement of my friend. When we lived together several years earlier, she had just severed a long, unfulfilling relationship with her boyfriend. She used to tell me that living at our address helped rebuild what had been broken down inside of her. So fast forward nearly three years, and what you will find is a person re-discovered, newly engaged to her perfect match, living... back at the same address (but now below in another unit) with her fiancé. Physical, emotional, and spiritual full circles unraveled before my eyes.

Circles remind us that when we start on a journey, any journey, when we return home (whatever that means, figuratively or literally), we are never the same. Life is cyclical. It is always changing, always moving, always transforming.

So the next time you are feeling stuck on the squareness of life, remember the circles. Next Monday, can be the start to your circular journey. And when you return, who knows where you might end up and who might be at your doorstep.

Growing In

Getting older is quite a peculiar experience. Our society frowns on age, constantly reinventing products and treatments that defy the aging process. But one night, while having an extremely overdue dinner with a good friend, I discovered some unexpected health insight in aging.

There are lots of fears around aging: forgetfulness, wrinkles, saggy skin... The list could go on. But as I sat across the table from a person who had known me for many years and caught up on the previous nearly three years of ups and downs in our lives, I could see, hear, and feel how much we had "grown in." Yes, we have continued to visually age, to grow up, but our minds and perspectives have grown into ourselves, and having the wisdom that comes only with age and experience is healthy.

In other cultures, becoming an elder is sacred. Gaining wisdom through life experiences and then sharing that wisdom with others is likened to being a high-powered leader, like having a seat in the Senate. So why is it that we constantly try to reverse aging? Of course, no one wants to lose a youthful appearance (or metabolism). But as I discovered that night, our conversation would have been much less meaningful had it happened three years earlier, two years earlier, or even a year earlier. Our conversation was rich with insight, humbling experiences, and most importantly, perspective that we had gained because of, not in spite of, getting farther and farther away from our high school graduation year.

So the next time you worry that you are getting older or already feel that you are old, remember that the wisdom we have, the insights we've gained, are because of our aging process.

Driving Me Healthy!

Driving has this amazing ability to create crazy behavior in seemingly normal people. Some people drive too fast, some too slow, others cut people off, run red lights, and roll through stop signs. It is very easy to bring out the worst in people by driving. But as I drove in the rain (which creates a heightened driver craziness), I found some unexpected health insights from being behind the wheel.

As I have mentioned before, driving can elicit quite a few unhealthy behaviors, primarily as a consequence of the stress that it induces. But the unexpected health in driving comes from what we all look at, gawk at, make fun of, and sometimes, are inspired by: bumper stickers. When I was stopped at a stoplight, I noticed the bumper sticker in front of me: "Practice Random Acts of Kindness." I had noticed this bumper sticker before, but every time I saw it, I was challenged to be a better person and having visual reminders to continually be better is healthy.

It is easy to get caught up in our own lives, our own agendas, all of the places we need to be, and all of the things we need to accomplish. When this happens (and it happens to all of us), we so easily miss what's right in front of us. So amazing little nudges like bumper stickers force us to remember where our focus should be. Now of course, we've all seen those bumper stickers that are a little outlandish, a little over the top, and some that are downright offensive. Even these are healthy because if nothing else, they give us a good laugh as we wonder, "Who in the world would put that on their car?"

So the next time you are driving, don't worry about the long traffic lights, ignore the slow driver in front of you, and forget about the person who just cut you off. Look at what messages you are given from the bumper ahead of you. Maybe it's exactly what needed to grab your attention that day.

Starting to Understand

"Well behaved women rarely make history." I love this saying. If you think about the people that have made some of the biggest impacts in history, it is not the meek and reserved. The people who are written into our history books are those who caused a rumble. They are forever known as the movers and shakers, refusing to settle for mediocrity. I discovered that unexpected health is rooted in empowerment when we take a stand.

There are lots of obvious healthfulness stemming from taking a stand: we gain respect for ourselves and value ourselves, our needs, and our desires in life, and the more we stand up for ourselves, the more we create our imprint in this world. But the unexpected health that arises from taking a stand is that when we put our foot down, we are not only empowering ourselves, we also empower others to do the same... And creating a movement of change is healthy.

As I have previously mentioned, I loved the movie *Invictus*. If you haven't seen it, cancel your plans for tonight, eat popcorn, and get wildly inspired by this film. Anyway, Nelson Mandela used empowerment to cause a movement toward peace and reconciliation. He empowered those around him, those considered "under" him, and as people felt that their opinions, wants, and desires mattered, the pulse of positive change started to beat stronger. Now of course, empowerment can also be used for great harm. Just as we will always remember Mandela, we will also never forget the abuse of power from a man named Hitler. But when our intentions, our morals, and the greatest good are at the forefront of our actions, we can be movers and shakers. We may never be typed into a history book, but in our community, in our family, in our circle of friends, we can create movement toward health.

So the next time you are prompted to stand up for your health and that of your fellow humans, remember that well behaved people rarely make history. Although you might feel uncomfortable putting your best foot forward and doing something not considered well behaved, standing up for change is healthy. And maybe your action can cause a chain reaction in others, maybe not. The more we take a stand, the more history we are making.

Choose Your Own Adventure Toward Health

My group of friends and I make a conscious effort to try new activities, go to new places, and experience new adventures, especially when we have something to celebrate. So for birthdays, holiday weekends, or just any old average day, we have collectively taken up rock climbing, snowshoeing, run groups, and on that day, hiking at a new location. We are all active, so it is very easy to buy in when one of us wants to try something new. And of course, that day was no exception.

The place we went to was beyond words... But I'll give you some anyway. We were surrounded by greenery that could have been in a movie. As we hiked up the seemingly endless stairs, we could see and hear the creek flowing down the side of the mountain, right next to the steps. At one point, the water spilled onto the stairway, creating an almost fountain-like effect. Once we made our way up to the hiking path, we turned the corner of one of the hillsides and immediately came face to face with creation so amazing we had to stop and take it in. Peaks and valleys, unbounded territory, and out further, what looked like sky was actually the ocean. None of us cared that we slopped through mud, getting our shoes and pants dirty. Nobody cared that we were hot and then cold, lost and then found. We collectively had an adventure. And as I was making the trek, I couldn't help but think about all the health that I was taking in: from the scenery to the fresh air to the company, I was inundated with health. But I also discovered a little unexpected health as well: the health we find in exploration.

When we push ourselves out of our comfort zones and explore new places, new experiences, new food, we are actually reversing the aging process. Now I know I have talked about how getting older is unexpectedly healthy, and it is. But reversing some of the negatives associated with getting older is also healthy. When we age (I am making a generalization here), we tend to gravitate toward consistency. I notice older people like to eat at the same time, have their get-togethers on the same days, even talk about the same topics. There is great ease in routine, in knowing. But when we branch out of our tree, we are reminded of all the beauty we are missing, and discovering beauty in life is healthy.

Routine is not a bad thing. In fact, I think we all do much better if we have it. But there is a difference between having routine in our daily lives and trapping ourselves in sameness. It is productive to schedule time in our days… It gives us direction. But to eat at the same restaurants, go to the same places, and even be with the same people limits our world to the knowns. I propose we challenge ourselves to the unknowns. As I discovered today, my unknown turned out to be one of the most gratifying, most health-filling experience I have had in nature.

So the next time you have the choice of a restaurant, an activity, even a destination, choose an unknown. You never know what beauty will be around the next bend.

Lucky Lessons

One of my favorite pastimes involves spending the day indoors, running the sport court floors in my jersey while playing in a volleyball tournament.

Whenever I play in these tournaments, I am immediately flooded with memories of my past playing days. I wake up early, pack about three shirts, two pairs of socks, snack foods, knee pads, and nowadays, a little Tiger Balm for my achy joints and muscles. I love the overcrowded gyms: backpacks, gym bags, lawn chairs, coolers, and of course, bags, carts, and baskets full of volleyballs strewn across the sports arena floors. In this way, I am a total gym rat at heart.

Once, as I was thoroughly enjoying my day full of sideouts and timeouts, I discovered some unexpected health insights about volleyball. Amidst the tremendous exercise, the teamwork and the experience, volleyball brings about a wealth of health with a little bit of luck. And feeling like you've got luck on your side is healthy.

Sports (in my case, volleyball) are often associated with luck. Players have lucky socks, lucky shirts, and lucky jockstraps (hopefully washed, but sometimes an unwashed jockstrap is lucky). Most players have some sort of pre- or post-game ritual: some eat the same breakfast before tournaments, others crack their knuckles, jump around, say a prayer. And for some reason, there is a belief that if players do the same routine, the same ritual, the end result is a big W-I-N. But the interesting part of these lucky rituals is that at some point we lose, and yet the rituals remain. If it was really lucky, wouldn't everyone win all the time?

The healthy aspect of luck is that luck, of whatever kind, stems from a belief. Thinking you have luck on your side gives you the belief, even if it is imagined, that everything is going to be okay. In volleyball, you switch sides every game. If a team wins on one side of the court, then loses on the other side, you better believe they will argue for the tie-breaking game to be played on the first side, because that's where the team won! It never fails. When the coin toss is called, odds are that the team who just lost would rather receive first (meaning they don't start serving) if it means they can have their winning side. Now most of the time, the sides are exactly the same. One side may have a weird glare or something like that, but all in all, there is no difference. What is different is the attitude that one side is luckier and will produce a win more than another.

What if we started thinking of ourselves as lucky in life? What if we started believing that our side of the court, our life, was the "it" spot, the winning side? I wonder if our circumstances would shift. I find that the more we think something is true, the more it is actualized as truth.

So the next time you think about being lucky (or not), expand the concept of luck beyond the roulette tables, beyond the that's-just-my-luck thinking, and beyond the winning side of the court. Luck can be whatever we believe in, so believe that luck is in everything!

This is Gutsy...

My rationale for writing this book has been to expand our definition of health, to create a larger pool for healthy experiences and practices to seep into our lives in some unexpected circumstances. If nothing else, it's another read to squeeze into your already busy life. Today, in the midst of trying on clothes, I discovered some very unexpected health in my dressing room.

Let me first clarify by saying that dressing rooms are not necessarily healthy. Actually, a dressing room (at least for a female) can be a torturous location. Three-way mirrors, bad lighting, and a stack full of clothes that don't quite fit can really tank a perfectly normal day. But in almost every dressing room is at least one mirror and in front of that mirror is you. As we "grow in," we are all faced with looking at ourselves, seeing with bad lighting and all who we are and what we have become. What I noticed one day while looking in the mirror was that my gut (and I use this word very purposefully) was more prominent than it used to be.

I used to pride myself on my abdominal muscles. Because of volleyball, my belly was in tip-top shape. But as my time on the court has lessened substantially, my core muscles have slowly dwindled, leaving a less-than-rock-solid gut.

But as I stood in the dressing room, I thought about how my bigger gut is more prominent because it has a larger, healthier role in my life. And appreciating ourselves for exactly as we are today is healthy.

Let me explain: you've all heard the sayings, "Go with your gut," "My gut feeling," "I have this gut instinct..." I have always had these gut moments but when I was younger, I ignored them. Now, I listen to the butterflies in my stomach. I emotionally examine the knots that form when I am anxious. I pay attention when I am sick to my stomach.

Our gut is our second heart. It tells us instinctively what we know (our intuition) but what our brains have yet to compartmentalize. Because of this, having a more visually present gut can actually be a very healthy reminder to pay attention. Now of course, excessively large bellies pose known health concerns, but a little extra padding around our second heart is not such a bad thing after all. The trouble is, one of the biggest targets of get-slim-quick programs is the belly. We are taught to crunch ourselves to abdominal agony. We do sit-ups by the hundreds, thousands... All of this is healthy, of course, because you can't have strong extremities without a solid core. But you can't have a strong sense of self without listening to your gut.

So the next time you pinch your gut, instead of thinking about how you need to slim down, appreciate the extra wisdom you are given from your belly's voice box.

Pardon the Interruption

The phone rings. The text message notification dings. The landline isn't answered so the cell phone rings. The inbox is bolded, indicating a new email is awaiting attention. A client walks in and needs an immediate answer. Does any of this sound familiar? We are inundated with communication needs. In person, online, all the time... How do we ever get anything done? Well sometimes, on a given day, we don't. Other days, an hour might go by without any interruptions. Those days are rare gems, and I'd like to dig up a few more of such peaceful times. But one day, in the midst of countless phone calls, discussions, needs, and agendas, I discovered some unexpected health while being interrupted.

Having disruptions in your day can be downright annoying. You lose your train of thought. You lose your place. You forget what the heck you are doing, where you are going, and what you needed to do. And at the end of the day, all of your interruptions just push back the day's tasks onto tomorrow, creating a snowball effect of work to be done that isn't getting done because you keep getting interrupted. That day was one of those days for me. I had a laundry list of to-do's, and I think at the end of the day, I accomplished two of approximately ten items on that list. As I was driving home from work, having had a very long, seemingly unproductive day, I thought about who interrupted me. And there it was, shiny and bright like my health *aha*'s always are: the people who I considered an interruption to my task list day were, I believe, put in front of me to help refocus my attention. And getting our focus adjusted is healthy.

As I have mentioned before, I can be a little bit of a dreamer. I can think big, bigger, huge! At times, this is necessary to expand. At other times, when tediousness is needed, I can get overwhelmed with the details. That day was one of those dream-big days. My mind was infiltrated with ideas, opportunities, and awareness about my business. But specific people came waltzing through the door or called me right as I started expending unneeded energy on a plan or vision that was not an immediate concern. They helped me focus... and refocus.

People keep us grounded, especially us dreamers. Others can see what is oftentimes a blindside for us. I find that those who tend to interrupt us the most (kids come to mind here) are some of the best teachers for us. They tug on the bottom of our shirts, trying to redirect our vision, to get our attention. The people who crossed my path on that day showed me where my focus should be. I believe people very intentionally show up in our lives when we need their perspective, their guidance, even their interruption.

So the next time you feel bombarded by people from all communication outlets, try not to focus on the distraction. Focus on the healthy guidance that cell phones attached to our hips does not mean we always have to answer.

Treetop Talk

Trees are truly a magnificent sight. Their deep roots, their substantial trunk, and their array of colorful leaves and branches remind me of the profound beauty of nature. But they also remind me of the beauty of people. In the fall, trees take on a brilliance. Their orange, red, and yellow hues make a statement of presence. You don't walk by trees like this without taking a second look. In winter, on the other hand, trees are barren. Their once abundantly leaf-filled branches turn to seemingly wimpy twigs sprouting out from the trunk. I find that people can appear this way as well. I have looked at some and wondered if they felt alive inside because on the outside, they appeared lifeless. So as I stared off into the winter landscape, I discovered the unexpected health in trees.

Trees have all sorts of known health benefits: they bear nourishing fruit for us to eat, they give us shelter, and of course, they are a ready-made adventure for any youngster waiting to climb them. But the unexpected health insight about trees is rooted in their appearance during the winter months. After autumn, the leaves fall away, the branches turn brown, and the beauty of a tree *seems* to fade, making that tree exposed. In winter, a tree's core becomes the most relevant attribute of focus. But zeroing in on the core, the essence, of people (and all other living organisms) is healthy.

You hear a lot about a person's core. In fitness, you are encouraged to strengthen your core (often referred to as your "trunk" in pilates—coincidence?!). Personal trainers help you build your abdominal, back, and chest muscles in order to stabilize the rest of your outer limbs. People also refer to the core of a person; they talk about their character, their morals. In the winter, we, like the trees, have the opportunity to let our cores shine. Trees don't have a choice, their leafy nakedness is not something the trees can prevent. But we can easily hide who we really are by pretending to be what we think others want us to be. The interesting part of hiding our true essence is that our uniqueness is what makes us strong and rooted in this world. It is our trunk that digs in deep, allowing us to sway with the challenges that life blows our way without being uprooted. And when we live life from our core, we experience health that is ideal for us.

So the next time you feel that who you are is not worth embracing, take a look at the winter's scenery. The trees may be showing you that a little exposure is just what you need.

Newsworthy

You will rarely find me poring over the newspaper or watching the six o'clock news. I find that most of the topics considered newsworthy inject fear-based thinking and living.

I remember there was a time when no one wanted to open their mail because of anthrax. Then we were bombarded with the terrorizing news that birds were going to kill off mankind with the bird flu.

But one time, I was pleasantly surprised by the topic my local newspaper chose to write about, and because of that, I discovered unexpected health in the news. I caught a front-page article of one of my fellow colleagues, who is educating the public about the importance of a healthy home by using non-toxic, everyday cleaners like baking soda, lemon, and vinegar. What a refreshing topic to see in the headlines.

Now of course, the expected health benefit to this article is the topic being discussed. But receiving a visual reminder that you are on the right path for you is healthy. I have questioned how I would use the education I spent two and a half years studying. Where does holistic health education fit into our society? Evidently, it fits in on the front page of a newspaper section. Whenever I have doubts about my career path, I can look at this article and be reminded that what I have to say is newsworthy. It is worth a two-page spread in a major newspaper. If you are questioning where you are but are passionate about what you are doing, look for those signs gently encouraging you to keep going. When we are questioned about our path, we can look for the answers.

Too often we are infiltrated with negativity. Our ears and eyes are inundated with depressing news about murders, child abductions, and celebrity sex scandals. Leaders and heroes of the American public topple off their pedestals by the dozens. And of course, the news is there to cover it all: we see pictures, hear stories, see rap sheets, because "if it bleeds, it leads," right? Let's change that. I propose we inundate our local news organizations with the positives we see in our world, in our daily life.

So the next time you see something healthy or experience something worth sharing, don't just tell your friend, your family, or your significant other. Share it. Write to your local newspaper, call the news station, write a blog. You just never know what someone else might also think is newsworthy. Let's change the old newspaper saying to "if it plants a seed, it leads." It's time for new growth. I'm Jaime Mathews, reporting from a location near you.

Finding Cheese in my Mouth Trap

I am a woman of many words. I am never one to pass up on giving my opinion. I jump at the chance to climb up on my soapbox and speak my mind and I definitely did not get an A in class for my quiet demeanor. Oh no, if you were to ask my junior high and high school teachers, coaches, and pretty much anyone else, they would tell you that Jaime was a little... let's just say "loud." Some might substitute "annoying" in there, but I prefer to be remembered by a more neutral term. But I was quietly humbled by the unexpected health I discovered in shutting up!

Now, let me preface this by saying that it was not me who actually shut my trap. But I learned a good lesson in being the bigger person and remaining silent. There are lots of healthy aspects that result from speaking your truth: you remain honest to yourself and to others, you empower yourself by standing up for what you believe, and of course, we have all heard the devastating stories of children, battered women, minority groups, etc., being mistreated and remaining silent. But sometimes (actually oftentimes), there is a quiet wisdom that surfaces in the silence, and tapping into wisdom of all volumes is healthy.

When we better filter our voice boxes, we practice wisdom. There is wisdom in speaking our truth. And there is wisdom in sitting back and letting others learn their own lessons, in their own time. I find that when I feel the incessant need to rattle off my thoughts, I am trying to control. I am attempting (even if my intentions are good) to make someone do what I think is best for them. How do I know what is best for someone? I barely know what's best for me sometimes!

So the next time you feel your tongue about to tango out a litany of words, consider taking the road less travelled and keep your mouth shut! It's amazing to sit back and see how life very quietly unfolds, especially when you let go of the reins.

The Gift of Surprise

One weekend I spent some much needed relaxation up in the mountains with eight of my closest friends. Over the years, we have become an incredible travel group. We could, and sometimes did, tell stories of past trips until the early hours of the morning. We have spent a good amount of time laughing until our stomachs hurt, and have definitely created some needed joy in each other's lives. In this way, we are vitally healthy to each other. But on that mountain trip, as I thought that a day could not possibly get any healthier (let's see, that day consisted of bright, warm sunshine and a fantastic day skiing), I found some unexpected health in surprises.

Who doesn't love a good surprise? As kids, my brother and I would stay up late waiting for Santa Claus to come eat our homemade cookies and drink our milk. We were also waiting to see what he filled our stockings with. We would sneak out, grab our grandma's handmade stockings with our names on them and run into our rooms and dump our entire stash on the floor in front of our Mickey Mouse night-light. Yep, I remember it as if it were yesterday. As adults, we still love a good surprise. I think, even if we don't admit it, we still love the surprise of opening Christmas presents.

But what I realized on that day is that some of the most seemingly insignificant surprises can be just as profound as Old Saint Nick climbing down our chimneys on Christmas Eve. I find that we underestimate how much our presence, including our surprise entrances, can literally make a loved one's day or even one's weekend… And realizing how essential we are to each other is healthy.

I watched and listened to the reaction we all had when one of our friends came walking through the cabin doors that afternoon after we thought he had gone home. You could immediately feel the energy rise in the room. It was as if the group had been completed again. It's amazing how each and every person's dynamic in a group can positively affect the rest. And I find it a pleasant surprise to be the recipient of such a joyful welcome when I unexpectedly attend an event. We don't have to throw large-scale parties to make a surprise profound. We can create health in our loved ones and ourselves just by showing up and being present.

So the next time you don't think your presence is missed, that whether you go or not doesn't matter, think again. Watch for the reactions you get when you walk through the doors of a home filled with friends. I bet, at that moment, you will be surprised. Because your surprise, your presence, just created a house full of health.

Naming Health

As you know, my name is Jaime. As a child, I hated my name because the spelling always created confusion and often during the roll call on the first day of school, I would dread to hear my name called, "Hi-may Mitchell, are you here?" I would sheepishly reply, "Here," which would immediately prompt the response, "Oh, I guess your name is Jaime... It's spelled differently." Yes, thank you parents! Now, I love my name. I even love the spelling. One morning, while walking through the very accurately named Big Trees area, I thought about the unexpected health that spells out a name.

Names are very significant. Names forever stamp a meaning on an organism... And being remembered for something unique and special is healthy. People think long and hard when naming their children, their businesses, even their animals. As I walked that morning, I was introduced to a lively labradoodle named Buddy. Buddy was watching and following his human friend from house to car as his human was packing to leave. This name was so fitting for this fun-loving ball of fur. You could see what a good companion, a good buddy, this dog was to his human. It was not hard to see the health benefits of their friendship. At that moment, I wondered if his human understood the unexpected health benefit of choosing a specific name for his four-legged pal, that choosing that name was also fulfilling a need for a friend.

Further on my walk, I was surrounded with the peaceful solitude of a morning in the mountains. I heard running water, no doubt a result of the snow melt because of the amazingly sunny day we'd had the previous day. I heard an owl hooting, a squirrel barreling up a tree, and once in a while, I would hear a dog barking in the distance. I was surrounded by nature, earth, and majestic beauty.

As I was taking in all of nature's beauty, I thought about another name: Tara. The name in all of its spellings means "hillside." For some reason beyond my human comprehension, I thought about the tragic loss of a family friend's daughter named Tara. I didn't know her very well, so I found it peculiar that I thought of her that morning. But then I realized that she is in everything. Her very significant name and her time here on this planet are forever embedded in the beauty of our world, our hillside, our Earth, our Tara. It made me sad to think about all of her loved ones left behind to grieve her absence and at the same time, as I walked through the magic of this place, I thought of her and her name. I correlated the timeless beauty of my surroundings with her. I thought that when her loved ones are sad and miss her, maybe they too find some solace, some peace, in the natural scenery of Earth that her name evokes.

We don't know how much time we have here on this planet. We never know when we might gain a buddy or devastatingly lose a loved one. But we have the choice to make something of our name. We have the opportunity to live each day to its fullest, most healthy potential. So, if you haven't looked up the meaning of your name, or if you don't remember what your name means, read about it. Your parents named you for a reason, for a purpose. Live up to that purpose.

My name means "supplanter," which means "to replace, to succeed." I plan to live up to my name in the healthiest way possible. I challenge you to do the same.

So the next time you are called on to name a pet or a child, think about it wisely. You are giving them an intimate piece of their identity.

MPH: Miles Per Health

Following a weekend of sunshine and snow, I returned to the Bay Area, greeted by more sunny skies and a warm sixty-five-degree day. After throwing a load of laundry in the wash, a few of my buddies and I decided that we just couldn't pass up on the opportunity to get a little exercise outdoors. So we fastened our helmets, velcroed our bike shoes, and away we went for a bike ride. At this point, I could talk about the health aspects of bike riding, of which there are lots, but I'm sure you already know them. I could also press Play on my song and dance about how the sun shines health on us. But while cruising at a challenging seventeen miles per hour, with the wind in my face, bugs in my teeth, and an already sore rump, I discovered the unexpected health in traveling without a car.

There are many known health benefits to leaving the car keys and opting for another form of transportation. The word exercise stands out. The savings on gas, the environment and our sanity are other obvious health bonuses. But the unexpected health that comes from leaving your car in the driveway for a day (or even an hour) is that when you unfasten yourself from your box on wheels, you open yourself up to the world around you, and giving and receiving fuel from other organisms is healthy.

On a nearly hour-long jaunt on my bike, I felt healthy physically, mentally, and emotionally. My body felt healthy from the workout, my mind felt rejuvenated by the scenery, my spirit felt alive with energy from the sun. I felt connected to my friends riding with me, to the strangers passing by me, and to the cars whizzing around me. When I am driving, I am confined to a four-wheeled configuration of windows and doors that literally block me from others (except when I have my windows down and sunroof open, which as all of you know, I often do!). Yes, cars keep dangerous objects from hitting us, but they can also shield us from some much-needed connection. When we are abiding by the speed limit while inside our cars, we can miss what takes place when we slow down and experience life outside of them.

So the next time you need to run an errand nearby, opt out of taking the car. Instead, grab your walking shoes, your bike, or even your skateboard, and experience a little health from your window-free mode of transportation: yourself.

Recharged for Health

On another beautiful afternoon, I felt the urge to soak up a little sun, so I left work a little early, drove home (windows down and sunroof open, of course!), changed my clothes to a tank top and shorts to make sure my skin would feel the warmth of the day, and off I went up to my neighborhood open space. That hike did not include a lost dog in its adventure, but I did have what I thought to be a small setback. However, after an hour on a dirt path between the rolling hills and the green, overgrown grass, I discovered that my so-called setback was actually my unexpected health insight for the day: the health that recharges us when our batteries are dead.

As soon as I was outdoors, I felt the desire to run. Now, this desire does not happen often, so when I feel it, it is essential I act on it. For that reason, I keep music in my car just in case I ever need musical inspiration to keep my legs moving. Well on that day, as soon as I hit the ground running, my music was nowhere to be heard. After pushing the Play button, and then pushing it harder (you know, if you push a button extra hard it's supposed to work, right?!)... Nothing. So, I was left to trek around huffing and puffing to no music. But what I lost in melodies, I gained in mindfulness, and being given the opportunity to tune in is healthy.

Music has a substantial amount of health benefits, but silence is also booming with health. Because my battery life had reached its capacity, I was forced to listen to the music of my surroundings. I listened to wild and domesticated animals. I heard conversations between people, between people and their animals (those are always entertaining... including my own!), and between my mind and my heart. When I have no other distractions, I can tune in to my internal communication. Those quiet nudges that I can easily disregard because I'm noise-distracted, are voluminous when my world is without noise. But sometimes, fate has to step in to force me to pay attention. On that afternoon, fate came in through low battery.

So the next time you freak out because a musical vessel of choice runs out of battery life, consider it a blessing in disguise. When your battery life is depleted, you have the opportunity to recharge your internal life.

Words of Wisdom

I. Love. Words. I love the written word. I can't get enough of a play on words (I'll get back to this later). I love acronyms, synonyms, action verbs and adjectives. I love literal stories and metaphorical insights. As I worked with words both written and spoken, I discovered how unexpected health is spelled out when we don't take words so literally.

I'm quite certain there are numerous ways that words in literal form are healthy: being told "I love you" promotes healthy connection and being congratulated encourages self-esteem. But the unexpected health insight from words is how expanded our perspective can become when we throw out the dictionary and get a little wordy.

I was once given a gift. Prepare for some play on words: the gift I received did not come wrapped in pretty paper or neatly tucked in an overpriced gift bag. The gift I received was the gift of collaboration. Try wrapping *that* and putting it under the Christmas tree! Collaboration, although wildly anticlimactic when compared to the highly popular blue Tiffany's box, is a gift that keeps on giving… and receiving. When you collaborate, you are helping equip others with a lifetime of tools for health and success. This is a gift that will not eventually tarnish. The gift of collaboration brings me to another healthy play on words that correlates with gifts: when someone asks me what gift I want, I like to say I prefer presence, not presents. Give me the gift of connection and activity, rather than trinkets and knick-knacks.

The spoken word can so easily be taken out of context. Or we can take words so literally that we miss what's really being said. I prefer practicing the art of taking words at more than face value and focusing on what is really being said behind the subject and verb.

So the next time you are listening, talking, or reading, try expanding your dictionary definition of the words you hear. You never know what healthy insights you might retain when you hear. When you hear, you're here, so be present to the gifts words give you.

Good Night Equals Good Health

I have always loved getting my zzz's. I've never been one to sleep past eight, but I do require seven to eight hours of sleep every night… That is, for optimal functioning. And my sleeping hours have always been significant as well, but that goes for most people. I do best when I go to sleep around 10 or 11 p.m., and wake up between 6:30 and 7 a.m. But one time, as my alarm clock echoed through the silence of my bedroom at a nearly-middle-of-the-night time of 4:30 a.m., I quickly realized the unexpected health that results with normal sleep.

Now of course, there are lots of known health benefits from counting sheep at a relatively early time in the night: greater probability of falling into REM sleep (Rapid Eye Movement, or deep sleep), greater chance of maintaining an optimal circadian rhythm, much stronger chance of waking up on the right side of the bed in the morning. But the unexpected health knowledge gained from a proper night's sleep is that sleep between the hours of ten in the evening and seven in the morning creates warmth, and feeling warmth both physically and emotionally is healthy.

Have you ever noticed when you are abnormally tired that your body literally feels cold? I notice that not only are my extremities cold, but my mind feels a little cooler as well. When we are sleep-deprived, the world looks a little bleaker, a little darker, a little colder. I find that everything inside me functions a little less healthfully when I am overly tired. I can overreact, misunderstand, and am quicker to anger and slower to forgive... All from a little lack of sleepy time.

So the next time you find yourself getting a little cranky, ask yourself if you got enough sleep. Of course, there are times when we are not going to get adequate sleep (having children comes to mind), and there is nothing we can do about that except adapt. But whenever possible, make sleep between optimal hours a priority. The world will look a lot brighter and feel a lot warmer when you do.

De-Funked Fridays

Previously, I talked about the wonderfully healthy benefits of Mondays. You remember: Mondays jumpstart your week. They are the perfect days for goal setting and go-getting. Well this time, I am happy to sing the praises and the unexpected health that lands on Fridays.

I'm sure you can think of a million ways Fridays are healthy: it's the start of the weekend, which can signify fun, relaxation, and rejuvenation. Fridays can start adventures, end work stress, and alleviate the workweek blues. But the unexpected health that occurs on this day is that I have dubbed Fridays as de-funk days. As Mondays warrant a desire to jumpstart the week, Fridays have a sneaky way of pulling you out of weeks gone wrong... And knowing that you have a way and a day to unwind is healthy.

It is easy to get overwhelmed and uninspired by Friday. We get discouraging news; we think we aren't doing enough; we leave our offices with piles of paperwork for Monday. But Fridays, especially around five in the afternoon, have this healthy way of making us forget, if even just for a weekend. Fridays are a time to gather with friends, relax with a movie, or get away (literally and figuratively). All of our problems may still be waiting for us come Sunday evening or Monday morning, but when it's Friday, all other stressors are more easily shelved.

So the next time you feel a little over-extended and under-appreciated, hold out for Friday. There is always an end to hardship... And oftentimes it's waiting for us at the end of the week.

Sore Winner

I am not as young as I used to be. My body told me that after a long volleyball tournament, when I walked slowly and sorely to my car. My shoulders were stiff from hitting all day, my back was tired from contorting myself in an attempt to dig a ball or hit an off-set, and my legs were like Jell-O from jumping to block and to hit. This body of mine felt a lot older than its actual age. As I hobbled up my stairs, it dawned on me that there is unexpected health masked in the odor of Tiger Balm and bound tightly in our aching and aging muscles when we are sore.

I know, it's hard to believe that there could be any health in stiff joints, achy muscles, and knotted backs. But there is! Being sore (or having any nearly debilitating physical ailment) forces us to pamper ourselves, and taking a little extra nurturing me-time is healthy. As I have stated time and time again, we live in an oftentimes painful world. We push ourselves to the limits, rarely taking the much-needed TLC essential to live our healthiest and most sustainable life. But when we do push ourselves past our limits, we come to a crossroads: do we keep pushing to the point of exhaustion, possibly inflicting permanent damage on our bodies? Or do we listen to our throbbing muscles and give ourselves a time out? I chose to take a big, fat T.O. that evening. I walked through the door, threw my gym bag on my bed, drew myself a hot bath with Dead Sea salts (great for sore muscles and joints), lit a candle and lathered a facial mask on my skin... And there I soaked. I didn't come home and immediately start unpacking my bag, making dinner, or cleaning up. Nope. I sank deep into my tub, relaxing my body after a physically taxing day, while giving my mind a little R&R after a busy week.

When we are sore from physical activity or pained from emotional stress, we are taught to work through the pain, right? As athletes, we learn to play harder, to stop at nothing. I get that. I was taught that. I tend to live my life that way. But sometimes, when we can't see the fast track we are quickly speeding down, our bodies will pull our own emergency brake, forcing us to stop, slow down, and take care of the only precious physical body we have on this planet.

So the next time you physically or emotionally tire yourself out, take the road less traveled. Give yourself a time out and take care of yourself. Your mind and definitely your body will thank you for it. As I sat typing away on my laptop, I could already feel my muscles loosening, my tension unraveling, and my mind relaxing... And I had my soreness to thank for that.

Giving Homework an A+ for Health

I spent a lot of time in school. My most recent school days were during my graduate program. My schedule was always pretty packed. I would work Monday through Friday until the afternoon and then head to classes at night. Sometimes I would have multiple night classes per week, three, sometimes four classes per quarter. On top of actual class time, I had endless amounts of homework. Weekends would arrive and constantly lingering over my plans was the paper, presentation, or program I had due the following week. Even though I loved what I was studying, at the end of the day, homework is homework. But once, after being the educator of a class instead of the educated, I found the unexpected health assigned to a little bit of homework.

Homework has all sorts of personal health benefits: you can earn a degree (or many), you gain insight into a field you may know little about, you learn how to work in groups, how to organize your time, and how to adhere to deadlines, and if nothing else, you may be able to answer a few more questions during a mean game of Trivial Pursuit. But the unexpected health you gain from being graded is that you now have tools to then share with others. All of your hard work, time, and money can be translated into both personal growth and community empowerment... And learning and sharing tools from all walks of life is healthy.

I happened to have learned tools for empowering others toward healthy living. That was my area of study. But I have gained countless amounts of helpful insight and knowledge from those in other walks of life: I have learned marketing and collateral design tricks of the trade from my creative friends and colleagues. I have been educated about marketing and business practices from business owners. My mind continues to expand from learning teaching techniques from my teacher friends. All of our knowledge about all of our varying areas of expertise are essential for us to grow in and expand out.

So the next time you question whether you have something to offer, whether your insight or opinion matters, or whether you should waste your time doing the homework of life (both graded and not), remember that we need each other. We must learn from each other, by each other, and with each other. If I ever get to a place in my life when I think I have learned it all, or even enough, I will immediately sign myself up for another class and another bout of homework assignments because I have obviously not learned one of the most fundamental lessons: life is not about arriving at a destination, it really is all about the journey.

Televised Health

I am not one to sit around and watch TV. I am uninterested in almost everything aired on cable. But as I plopped on the couch and turned on the tube, I found unexpected health appearing in advertising, sitcom, and reality form while watching television.

Now just to clarify, I am not advocating turning in your bike for a new eighty-inch plasma. I in no way think that watching TV should be your new hobby. But I do find that sometimes a little vegging out is necessary. Television programs and commercials (especially on Superbowl Sunday) can be quite hysterical at times, and laughing, however and at whatever possible, is healthy. Laughing causes us to release feel-good chemicals called endorphins. Being able to chuckle relaxes muscles, eases tension, and lifts our mood. Laughing out loud increases our immune functioning. And if nothing else, TV definitely makes us laugh.

I get a kick out of all the reality shows on TV these days. *The Bachelor*, *Dancing with the Stars*, *American Idol*... Every time you change the channel, there is a new reality show that is as far from realistic as an Ashton Kutcher movie. But however unrealistic, they can be really funny.

It is so easy to take life too seriously. We can dwell on all of our hardships, all of our stressors, and our endless to-do lists. For that reason (and it may be one of the only reasons), TV is healthy. A little time checking out of our hectic lives can actually be a very beneficial time to remind ourselves to lighten up. When we are able to check out of our craziness if even for an episode, we allow ourselves a healthy diversion.

So the next time you are teetering between working an extra half hour or calling it a day, consider a little laughing time, even a little TV time, a worthwhile use of time. If nothing else, watching these endless unrealistic reality shows might make you feel a little better about your own life.

Four Eyes on Health

I have a confession to make. When I was younger, I used to make fun of people who wore glasses. Yes, I called people "four eyes," and I'm sure the word "nerd" came out a time or two. I'm not proud. I was particularly *not* proud when I had to start wearing glasses in the fourth grade. Aah, life is always so humbling, isn't it?

Of course, I wore my glasses as little as possible, even playing sports without vision aid. In fact, it wasn't until after I graduated college that I actually got fitted for contacts and now I wear them religiously. But let's get back to the glasses. While watching a documentary on forgiveness, I discovered the multiple uses and of course, unexpected health, that's found behind the lenses of glasses.

I'm sure I don't need to tell you about the known health benefits of glasses: sunglasses shield your eyes from the nearly blinding rays of the sun. Glasses help you see more clearly. A good pair of shades can block your peepers from objects in the air. But the unexpected health that refreshingly appears in a pair of spectacles is that glasses create a different view and seeing a person or experience in a different light is healthy.

While watching that documentary, I learned how teachers

in Northern Ireland are using visuals (and metaphors) to teach children forgiveness. After a child would tell a story about someone who hurt them, they were asked to put on their "forgiveness glasses," and then say something good about that same person. In literally a few seconds, a child was able to distinguish a person's hurtful act from the person themselves. What a powerful vision of health. What if we were able to use our reading glasses, bifocals, and sunglasses to help us see more than our naked eyes are capable of? What if when we put on our black-, brown-, or orange-shaded glasses we could actually see something positive in those who have hurt us?

It is so easy to hold on to resentment, anger, and sadness when someone hurts us. It's hard to forgive. But then I think about times like the Troubles in Northern Ireland and I wonder how a family whose father or son was killed would be able to forgive. How would you teach a fatherless child how to forgive? There are so many objects we have in our daily life that we interpret so literally, like glasses. But what a great gift to realize that something so simple, so prevalent in all of our lives, can actually be used as a healing tool.

So the next time you reach for your slick pair of shades or your reading glasses, remember that your glasses have many purposes. Let your glasses block out the harm... But allow them also to let in the light that appears when we see others with different eyes.

Pediatric Health

This may not be the most obvious bit of unexpected health insight that I have ever written. There may be no new revelations except for my own. I imagine that for all you parents reading this, I am not telling you something you don't already know. But while spending some auntie-niece time during a hike, I discovered some unexpected health that is born in children.

Children are healthy for us wound-up adults for many reasons: kids keep us grounded, children force us to grow up and be adults, and youngsters encourage us to change family dynamics so that negative patterns of the past are hopefully not repeated. But the unexpected health that children gift our lives with is found imprinted in their steps.

Let's face it, children walk slowly. You've all seen this visual: a hurried parent nearly dragging their child behind them because the poor kid can't keep up with an adult pace. Kids literally can't keep up. I've noticed that we make children speed up in all areas of their little lives. We sign them up for any and every sports league possible. We've harnessed our children with leashes so we don't lose them. We plop them in baby joggers and push them along during our runs. I'm not saying sports leagues and baby joggers are a bad thing, but while walking with my niece, I found that when we actually slow down to a child's pace, we catch a glimmer of so much more... And seeing the beauty (and health) in the small things is healthy.

On our muddy excursion outdoors, my niece pointed out every (and I am not exaggerating here!) hole in the vast earth around us. She would floppily run with her little pink mud boots on, stop and gasp as if she had just found buried treasure, and shriek out that she had found another hole. I have never, in probably all my life, noticed these little squirrel holes, and I have walked, hiked, and ran in that space for years. Later, we actually picked wildflowers. Who does that anymore? Then, we rubbed our hands through the mud and then used the wet blades of grass as sanitary wipes to clean them. How often do we allow ourselves, or even our kids, to have such unadulterated, seemingly unsanitary fun?

So the next time you are given the opportunity to spend time with a kid, take it as a challenge to rediscover the beauty of seeing the world with child-like wonder. Kids are so incredibly innocent. Adults are so easily hardened. When I think about what kind of mom I continue to strive to be, I realized that although I want to teach my children morals, beliefs, and a good sense of self, I want to be sure to soak up what my children will undoubtedly teach me. To stop and notice the details, to pick wildflowers and give them to loved ones, and to experience the earth with wild curiosity. As we grow in, may we become more like the innocent children we once were.

Taking Health Through the Spin Cycle

Laundry is not my favorite task. But after a while, the overflowing laundry basket can no longer be ignored. So as I scooped up my pile of dirty clothes, threw them in the washer with some detergent, and closed the lid, I thought about the unexpected health that cycles through our life when we do the wash.

Now for those of you with large families, you may have a very hard time seeing any health piled in your endless loads of laundry. But when we do the wash, whether for ourselves or for our family, we are given the opportunity to clean off all of life's little messes... And knowing that we can start again fresh and clean is healthy.

If I didn't have a washer and dryer (or at least a washer), who knows how many muddy adventures I might skip out on. But my washer allows me to play with reckless abandon because I know that I can easily remedy my messy problem.

We Americans have so many luxuries plugged into our lives and yet we seem to be some of the most uptight people on the planet. How can we have so much readily available to us and at the same time be wound up like a cuckoo clock?

Most of us don't have to take our clothes down to the nearest river to wash them. We have the opportunity to get a little dirty, to stomp through the mud and play in the rain. We can just throw our clothes in our washer.

So the next time you are worried about getting your clothes wet, your hands dirty, or your shoes stained, don't! Just live a little. That's what the OxiCleans, Bleach Pens, and Colorguards of the world were created for.

Spoonful of Frustration

I am no Mary Poppins. A spoonful of sugar does nothing for my physical health, my mental health, or my state of mind. Although I still love this sixties classic and Mary Poppins's school of thought is healthy in its own way, I actually found a spoonful of my own unexpected health today from getting mad.

Yes, getting mad is very uncharacteristic for that iconic British nanny. But just as being sugary sweet is healthy for some experiences, getting downright pissed off is completely necessary for others... And understanding that you don't always have to be perfectly composed is healthy. Sometimes, the healthiest response you can have is to get mad.

I find that getting mad pushes us to a crossroads, and crossroads of all kinds are positive places to be. When we arrive at a crossroads in our lives, whether it be a career decision, a relationship decision, or even a driving decision, we are presented with options. Crossroads force us to make a decision that will undoubtedly change the course of our path, and the very fact of coming to a crossroads means that a decision needs to be made. From an emotional standpoint, I find we often don't make decisions until we actually come to these forks in the road... And these often come when we get fed up and angry.

I have a hard time really getting angry. I try and maintain my cool as often as I can, but I have found that getting mad has propelled me to make some very healthy decisions in my life, decisions I would probably never have made if life stayed monotonous, free of annoying situations and frustrating people.

So the next time you feel yourself getting perturbed, don't worry about maintaining Mary Poppins composure. It's okay to get angry. In fact, it's necessary. If you are angry and fed up, rest assured that a little healthy change is coming your way.

Drops of Health

Rainy days are often not my favorite. I do not enjoy wet pant legs when they drag on the watery ground, wiry, frizzy hair is not my best look, and forget about keeping your floors clean if you have a dog. But as I walked from my car to the house on a rainy and dreary day, I was startled by the unexpected health that pours on us with drips of rain.

As I hurried to get out of the dark, open sky and under the shelter of my house overhang, I was doused with a raindrop the size of a grape... At least, that's what it felt like. The bangs that I had actually taken the time to fix this morning immediately shriveled into the awkward swirl on my forehead that I try so desperately to straighten out. (Curly hair is much easier to tame in the summer!) But, as soon as that drip hit my forehead, I literally jumped, and being jolted back to reality is healthy. But let me back up...

I woke up in a peculiar mood. I guess I woke up in a fog, so to speak. My mind was unclear, much like the experience of driving in the fog... You don't quite know what's going on or what's in front of you. I got up, got dressed and headed out to do my errands. Although I had read about mindfulness earlier in the morning, I was anything *but* paying attention. But then, like a bolt of lightning that rattles the Earth, I was struck with a raindrop... Well actually, it was a rain drip. The cold gush of water that fell on my face woke me up. I might have physically risen out of bed this morning, but I was very much asleep until Mother Nature decided I was not truly awake yet.

Getting wet from the rain can be annoying. But I find that it is also quite healthy... and healing. After being jolted by the drip, a slight smile came across my face because I knew something more and someone other than myself was trying to get my attention. And it worked.

So the next time you have an off day, remind yourself that it is perfectly okay to feel like life is a little strange. But when it's time to focus less on the strangeness and more on the beauty and opportunity, life has a funny way of waking us up. And sometimes, what wakes us up is anything but our alarm clocks.

Questioning Health

I ask a lot of questions. I would say that I have always been a searcher of answers. Throughout my quest for the truth, I have often heavily relied on external, non-human sources such as books, the internet, or even a good old-fashioned guess (hey, your guess is as good as mine, right!?). But sometimes, actually oftentimes, the best insights come from a little face-to-face Q&A. After numerous question, answer, and insight sessions, I discovered the unexpected health that turns question marks into exclamation points when we ask questions.

Now, asking questions reveals all sorts of obvious health benefits: you find answers to the painstaking questions you may have, or you may have a health question that is answered, enabling you to physically experience greater health. But the unexpected health in questions is that asking questions means we feel empowered enough, healthy enough, to deserve to know the truth, and understanding our worth as individuals is healthy.

Asking questions is a humbling experience at times, because it means that we don't have all the answers. For someone who is somewhat proud at times in my life, you can imagine how difficult this has been for me. But as I have grown in, I have shelved my pride and raised my hand (well let's be honest, I never did that very well, even in school), asking any and every question I possibly could because what I don't ask, I don't know.

Not knowing is often associated with the commonly used phrase "in the dark." We call these dark dwellers "clueless," "checked out," and a whole slew of statements that point out their lack of knowledge or even common sense. When I think of being in the dark, I immediately look for light, because to be honest, I don't really like the dark very much. When we are in the dark, we have a hard time focusing on anything, even things that are right in front of us. Not asking questions is a lot like that. When we refrain from knowing more, we are left in the dark, unaware. But when we choose to know more, ask more, we are allowing ourselves to be enlightened.

So the next time you fret over asking a question or not, raise your hand, blurt it out, do whatever you need to do to find out more. Even if your question leads to more questions, consider that your way of turning on the light in your world.

Feeling A Little Health Sick

I'm not going to lie: I pride myself on my above-average immune system. I eat lots of antioxidant foods (vitamin C and I are good friends), drink lots of water, and most days, get my seven to eight hours of sleep. But one dreary morning, I woke up a little under the weather. I wouldn't say I was actually sick, but I definitely didn't start the week fully charged with energy. But as I thought a bit about why I might be feeling a little less than optimal, I diagnosed myself with a little unexpected health in being sick.

Being sick allows us to take care of ourselves. We sleep a little more, rest a little more, drink a little more tea, and hopefully eat a little less junk food. But the unexpected health that creates the perfect medicine is that sickness allows us to create our own health... And becoming the healers of our own bodies is healthy.

You've probably heard the saying, "Healer, heal thyself." Well, this is not just meant for those with an MD at the end of their names. We are all healers in our own way, in our own lives. When our bodies react to exhaustion, to a virus, to an allergy, we are given the opportunity to do a little investigative self-reporting. As I woke up feeling a little under the weather, I immediately began the journey toward discovering what my body might be telling me. What I discovered is that I may have an allergy to my new bed pillows.

But I would never have discovered this health tidbit if I had not been forced to pay attention. As I have stated time and time again, we are busy little bees. It is easy to check out—out of our bodies, out of our minds, out of our internal knowing. Being under the weather or downright sick gives us permission to dig into ourselves, to find out what makes us healthy and what makes us sick. Of course, not all remedies can come from within. That's why doctors are also so valuable. But there are times when, if we pay just a little more attention to ourselves, we can find out what's going on.

So the next time you are unwell, consider it your wellness opportunity to get to know *you* a little more. You never know what factors might be making you sick in life... And what remedies might make you well. For me, I'm getting a new pillow.

Science Experience

Have you ever had a really great idea but nobody believed in you? Do you ever think to yourself, "Gosh, this is so great if only it could get into the hands of the right person?" I've had that thought many times in my life. Unfortunately, either those hands have never waved me down, or maybe, just maybe, my idea wasn't as fantastic, as mind blowing, as I had thought! Well one night, as I sat with total satisfaction watching healthy practices be proven measurably healthy, my double-blind experiment concluded that unexpected health occurs in science.

There was actually nothing double-blind about my experiment. Both eyes, ears, and my heart were completely open. But what I discovered was that although science has many known, textbook-cited health benefits (cures for a variety of diseases, research on genetics, smoking, and disease), the unexpected health proven in science comes from the results... And having tangible measurements of our health and life is healthy.

Now, let me be clear: when I say measurements, I am in no way talking numbers on the scales, which in and of itself, is not always a strong indicator of health. Nor am I referring to your BMI, your age, or your waist-to-hip ratio.

I am referring to your blood pressure. Those two little numbers (hopefully in the 120/80 range) are such powerful indicators of our health, wellbeing, and state of mind. On that night, I watched as researchers and scientists proved that the simple act of forgiveness can lower blood pressure, which of course, increases health.

We live in a culture of high pressure, high stress, and ultimately, high blood pressure. Hypertension affects countless Americans and those affected are becoming younger and younger. But blood pressure medication can have a detrimental effect on our physical body. So I wonder what our lives would be like if we used a practice such as forgiveness to treat hypertension. What would our drug companies do if we opted out of our prescriptions and instead picked up refills of love, forgiveness, and humanity? I am not saying that medication is unnecessary, but I do wonder what kind of world we would live in if running to the drug store wasn't our first remedy option.

So the next time you take your blood pressure medication, consider the proven scientific data on the most all-natural, non-toxic, organic form of medication on the market for hypertension—forgiveness. Seems like a wonderful compliment to your prescription. No healthcare plan needed.

Nightlife

10:56 p.m.: I was in silence. No music, no phone calls, and no TV. I was quietly lying in my bed, my favorite place to reflect upon and write about my adventures with unexpected health. But wait, a noise... A very loud, booming noise began piercing the quietness of the night. In fact, I recalled hearing this obnoxious noise the previous night! What the heck was anyone doing to make such a ruckus at that hour... On a Wednesday? I listened a little closer and discovered that that noise heard 'round the world (or just my neighborhood) was none other than a jack hammer... Yep, you read that correctly. At 11 p.m. on a Wednesday, jack hammers were puncturing our streets.

So of course, this obnoxiously distracting noise made me think. How could I possibly find health in this? Well, drumroll please... I chiseled my way toward finding the unexpected health that breaks up the silence with night work.

That night, as I lay there listening to the road construction taking place at that hour, I was reminded that opportunity is out there.... And knowing that there is a light at the end of any tunnel is healthy. Night work of any kind demonstrates that movement is still happening. In fact, there is so much movement that some of our movement carriers (like our roads) must be worked on in the wee hours of the night. On that night, someone had work jackhammering a street apart—or whatever else they were making all this noise for. What a bittersweet sound to be echoing off my otherwise quiet surroundings. Although I may have been kept awake, someone else was making enough money to put food on their family's table.

11:09 p.m.: The jack hammer was still breaking up cement. I heard a large construction truck backing up. You know how I knew it was backing up? By yet another noisy *beep, beep, beep* sound of the truck's reverse. What this meant (besides the fact that I was seriously considering relocating to the country at that point!) is that there were at least *two* jobs being done at that moment, and at least two people being compensated for contributing to society.

Of course, I would have loved to fall asleep to the sounds of crickets, or wind, or the ocean. But the city noise is a sweet little reminder that we are still moving, cities are expanding and our tides are constantly changing.

So the next time you are awakened to the early morning street workers, the late-night construction crew or the mid-afternoon renovation, remember that although they may be bothersome personally, they are expansive collectively. And if nothing else...

11:29 p.m.: Note to self—buy earplugs.

A Little Hair Health

If you haven't noticed yet, I really do love a good play on words. So let's *highlight* some important concepts I discovered, some unexpected health, if you will, while getting my hair done.

Now, there are lots of reasons that getting your hair done is healthy: cutting off dead ends to allow for new growth, transforming your look, which can boost your confidence, and of course, your hair follicles get a little TLC from those heavenly scalp massages. But the unexpected health that gets processed with your color is that as you are visually seeing your hair change, you have the opportunity to watch as those around you are changed as well.

I used to own a hair salon. For over six years, I sat behind the desk and watched clients come and go, entering with much less confidence than when they left. But, as I sat in the chair getting my own very prematurely gray hair covered up, I was pleasantly flooded with information, opinions, and insight.

It is commonly assumed that hair salons are gossipy, and to be honest, I'm sure there has been more than one occasion that I have sat in a chair, foil in my hair, starting conversations with, "Well, I heard that…," or, "Oh, well did you hear..." I for one know that I am guilty of salon chair gossip. But one day when I became acutely aware that I wanted positivity to come flying out of my mouth instead of gossip, I noticed that those around me were all very positive as well... And being witness to positive creating positive is healthy. In fact, not only did I have conversation after conversation about healthy topics, the entire energy of the salon was fantastic! I talked with the stylists, listening to the very humanitarian ways that they wanted to give back, to pay it forward. I talked with clients about the joy they receive from watching a good movie with their family or nestling up with a good book.

It is easy to expect experiences, people, and situations to be a certain way if society (I use this term loosely) tells us so. But what a treat to discover that we can and do create our reality. Now, I'm not saying this in a condemning way. I do not think that people who have illnesses or disease or experienced tragedy have brought these on themselves. But I do find that expecting greatness can in fact manifest some pretty cool experiences.

So the next time you are getting your hair done, remember to keep your eyes, your ears, and especially your heart open. You never know how you could be positively blown away by more than a hair dryer. Go ahead and cover up the gray, but expose the greatness.

Daily Health

"If you have made mistakes, even serious ones, there is always another chance for you. What we call failure is not the falling down but the staying down." — Mary Pickford

This daily thought was the first thing to greet me when I opened my email one morning. I set myself up to receive a thought of the day, every day (from Real Simple Magazine, in case any of you are wondering—a magazine that I highly recommend). I love starting my morning with a positive thought, a motivational saying, or some words of wisdom. It immediately makes me think, if only for a moment, about the goodness in life... And having continual reminders about the good in this lifetime, instead of focusing on the bad, is healthy.

Now of course, there are a plethora of reasons that daily thoughts are healthy: they can shift an otherwise negative mindset, inspirational sayings can lift our mood, and these little nuggets of truth can give us hope when we feel that our lives are failing. But the unexpected health about daily thoughts is that they teach us the fundamental truth about quality. These daily thoughts I receive are never more than a couple of sentences long, but in those perfectly arranged subjects and verbs are some of the most profound, most thought-provoking insights I could ever read.

I am not a short-and-sweet kind of writer and that's okay. But I am reminded daily of the importance of "less is more," that quality often trumps quantity. Sometimes the most influential advice I have ever received has come from short-winded people. When there are fewer words to process, there are greater chances of retention.

So the next time you are about to give advice, bend an ear, or offer your insight, remember that a little bit goes a long way. If you need a daily reminder of this (like I do), check out Real Simple. The name explains it all.

Digestive Health

In the wee hours of the night, I was awakened by pain. I tossed and turned, drank water, and then sat for nearly an hour, wondering what was going on inside my abdominal wall. Once I fell back asleep and then woke up when it was finally daylight, I thought about the unexpected health that grabs our attention with stomach aches.

Now, one might question how stomach aches can possibly be beneficial to our health. Well, stomach aches aren't expectedly healthy. In fact, they downright suck! But the unexpected health that arises when our stomach pains us is that when our stomach is upset, it is telling us that something is wrong... And having red flag verbalizers in our body is healthy.

The previous, I had eaten foods that I normally don't eat—at least not in excess. I had consumed more sugar and refined carbs than I like, but I did so anyway because of a celebratory event. Well, fast forward eight hours, and you will find me awake at 3:30 a.m., nursing a grumbling tummy. In the not-so-distant past, I ate more of these types of foods. But since choosing to fill my belly with more agreeable foods for my body, I now have a harder time reverting back to old habits.

As we further our understanding of ourselves, our bodies, and what is healthiest for us, individually, it becomes increasingly more difficult to be any other way. And when we participate in another way (like that day's self-inflicted sugar pain), we pay dearly. There is no turning back from health once we begin to experience how fantastic we feel when we are nourishing ourselves.

Dieters will say they are cheating when they eat something that their diet restricts them from. But I say, forget about cheating the diet. As we develop what gives us sustenance, we are not cheating some calorie-counting regime. We are inflicting pain, all kinds of pain, on ourselves.

So the next time you are surrounded by foods that you know do not agree with you or you get a stomachache, choose to nourish yourself. It doesn't mean you can't have what is being offered, it just means to know your limits and don't surpass them. Because when you do, you are only causing pain to yourself. Jenny Craig will not pay the price if you eat a disagreeable food... But your tummy will. Choose to be good to your belly.

Yappin' for Health

I was never the quietest kid on the block. In high school, I distinctly remember certain teachers not liking me because of what I would call my boisterous personality. Some might not have described me so gently, but I prefer to be wonderfully naïve to my most likely obnoxious behavior at times. I've just always had a lot to say and lacked the patience to wait my turn to speak. I guess that's why I am a writer... I can write and write and write and wait for nothing! It's funny how we intentionally and unintentionally choose career paths.

Anyway, back to the health. I have already talked about the health in silence, the insights that are gained when we refrain from speech. But after an email conversation with one of my closest friends, I discovered the unexpected health voiced through the lips of a yapper.

Yes, yapping (what my mom and I call "flapping our gums") contains a mouthful of unexpected health. Now of course, the immediate depiction of healthy yapping would be talk therapy. Also, talking through situations with friends and loved ones can alleviate misunderstandings. But the unexpected health in talking is that the more you have told your story to those around you, the greater reflection you will receive from others.

Let me explain: one time, I needed to bend the ear of my friend. My amazing friend, who has tirelessly listened to (or read about) my endless life stories, adventures, heart bursts and breaks, was again at the receiving end of my yapping (actually, typing). But what I found so health-filled and helpful was not only the words of encouragement she gave me. She knew my story. This friend has been through many ups and downs in my life. And because I am unable to keep quiet about my feelings, my thoughts, and my soapbox beliefs, she knows how to relate to me. She can bring up things I have said in the past, she can mirror to me what she has seen and heard... And having a friend hold a mirror to show you to you is healthy.

I am not proposing that we all become self-indulgent, excessive talkers. Nobody wants to be around someone like that! But I do find that it is important, actually essential, to open up. Keeping a lid on your emotions helps no one, especially not yourself. When we shut people out, we are taking away the opportunity for others to show up for us, to be a mirror when we need to see ourselves.

So the next time you feel the need to talk but don't want to be a burden to your loved ones, shut up that voice in your head and open your mouth and speak. I think you will be pleasantly surprised by the response.

Failing Health

I love inspirational books. I am a total sucker for quotes of the day, insights by Gandhi, and reflections from Emerson. I have been choked up from sayings uttered by anyone from Oprah to Simon Cowell (and as you all know, forget about TV commercials... Hand over the Kleenex!). Okay, Simon might be a stretch, but you get my point. I love to be inspired. And words inspire me.

A few words I read one day were particularly inspiring, but in an unexpected way. Eloquently written in Matthew and Terces Engelhart's book, *Sacred Commerce*, I gained profound insight, and unexpected health in failure.

The Engelharts, the co-creators and once owners of the wildly popular vegan restaurants in California, Cafe Gratitude, talk about failure a lot in this business practice book (which I highly recommend). They state that failure is essential. If we never failed, then we are playing the game of life too safe, which keeps us stuck in our comfort zone, inhibited from transformation, and ultimately, expansion, and of course, health. But our society teaches that failure is a bad thing, that if you fail at something, you are less whole. Not true! And realizing that every experience we have is supportive of our growth and change is healthy.

Failure is deeply embedded in our life's landscape at pivotal times. We can fail our driver's test (bummer if you are sixteen!). We can fail to get into a specific college. We can fail a college class. We can fail to get what we think is our dream job, our dream spouse, or our white-picket-fenced house with two point five kids. As we age, we can develop failing health, a memory that fails us, and failure to have bladder control. The failure list goes on and on throughout our life cycle. But what would happen if we thought of these moments of failure as an opportunity for transformation? I wonder how different we would feel about ourselves if we knew that for every seeming failure, a greater transformation is taking place.

On Tuesday nights, I have been attending a forgiveness class. Each week, we talk about how forgiveness can shift our mindset—or not, if we choose not to forgive. I know for myself that I have held onto more guilt than I would like in areas where I feel like I have failed. But as I begin to expand my understanding of failure, that it is necessary and (oh yeah!) not a bad thing, then I can take it easy on myself and others, and move forward.

So the next time you call yourself a failure or a loser, remember that to fail at something simply means that you are playing a high-risk game of transformation... And the winner of that kind of game will always be you!

A Little Corner of Health

Do you ever notice which area in a restaurant you prefer to sit in? I always like a corner. I like to have at least one area that is void of people, noise, a cross breeze, whatever. I always prefer a booth to a table. I will always opt for a quiet corner rather than squished in between two two-tops (that's restaurant lingo for two tables that fit two people). And I will always seat myself away from a crowd instead of right smack in the middle of one. Here's why: for the most part, when I go to dinner, I am going with one other person. And because of that, whether I'm meeting up with a close friend or loved one, I want to be able to engage with whomever I am with. So, because of this tabletop revelation tonight, I discovered a little unexpected health that occurs when, to make a little change to the *Dirty Dancing* movie phrase, you actually put "baby in the corner." Yes, we should all request our own little corner of health.

Now, there are lots of healthy reasons why people like to be placed in the hub of life: being in the center of the action can make us feel alive, that placement makes us feel a part of a larger community, and sometimes, the intimacy of a corner location can be intimidating, so we feel much safer (and I guess, much healthier) being in a crowd. But the unexpected health that's reserved at a corner table is that when we get away from the distractions of our world, we have the amazing capacity to connect at an enriched level with another person... And finding opportunities, anywhere, to connect with others at a heart level is healthy.

As I have reiterated before, we live loud lives. Even our restaurants, which were created for people to come together, to connect, have become massive halls with tall ceilings, echoing acoustics, and endless noise. If you go to parts of Europe, most of the restaurants you find are little quaint bistros or ristorantes that are dollhouse-sized compared to our Cheesecake Factory–filled nation. It's not that I dislike restaurants like Cheesecake Factory, but I do find that the level of depth between humans becomes harder and harder as the noise level is higher and higher.

One night, I had dinner with a very close friend. We have a habit of going to the same sushi restaurant and usually sit at the same table. This table is near the front of the restaurant, so we don't get the foot traffic or the breeze like other tables. But the healthiest aspect of this table is that, because of its placement, it allows us to dig right into our dinner and our conversation. We fill our bellies up with sushi while having enough peace and quiet to fill our minds and hearts with insights and inspiration.

So the next time you are planning a night out, think about the atmosphere you want to create. Yelp doesn't categorize eateries by their connection capacity, but sometimes, I wish they would. If you are looking for a little more than fine wining and dining, choose your restaurant wisely—and opt for the corner table.

Instant Health

I've talked in the past about the health benefits of waiting, the importance of holding back instead of plunging forward, how vital it is to observe rather than react. These are all qualities that I wish I possessed more of. I find that I do not think every single detail through. Some people would call that adventurous, courageous. Others would call it premature and careless. But as I was reminded of my often quick-reacting personality, I on-the-spot discovered the unexpected health in instant gratification.

Being instantly gratified is something Americans are very familiar with. We have quick fixes for just about anything, at any time, any day, and anywhere in the world. I can jump on the internet and get my hands on absolutely anything I want with the click of a button and probably have it delivered to my doorstep within forty-eight hours.

Now, the healthy aspects of instant gratification are actually hard to come by. Having everything so readily available makes us wait for nothing. In fact, the days of waiting are past tense. By the time you've read this sentence, you are probably already sick of having to wait for my punchline. Wait no longer: the unexpected health in instant gratification is that when we throw caution to the wind and act out of instinct (and I use this word choice very purposefully), we can cause a ripple effect of health for ourselves and others... And trusting our internal knowing is healthy.

Now, let me be clear: there is an enormous difference between acting from instinct and acting from insecurity. Instinctual action is a causal movement from a place of quiet, internal knowing. Insecure actions are those made from a place where our protective defenses take over our deeper sense of knowing what is most helpful for our lives. In other words, instant gratification from instinct is a much healthier option.

Let me give you an example: one night after having dinner together, my friend and I walked to our cars. Now, I had been carrying around a money tree in my car for a day or two. I had initially bought that tree for a friend who really needed some financial turnaround. But that night, I felt compelled to give this little plant away—immediately.

Now, you might chalk it up to trying to get rid of this green luck charm, but it wasn't. I just felt the immediate need to gratify some heart tug I was having; hence, a little instant gratification was in order. I, for some reason, needed to instantaneously gratify my heart's need to listen to myself... and I did.

Fast forward to the next day and the recipient of the money tree actually had a meeting today in which money was directly involved, and so my gift was quite fitting and timely. So my unceasing need to act immediately actually proved to be a need worth listening to. I could have easily saved the little plant for the original intended recipient, but I decided that it was more worthwhile to spend a little extra money and buy another plant. Pay it forward, right!?

It is easy to ignore our heart tugs, our inner sense of knowing. But when we listen, even to our moment of instant gratification, we can experience a little voice telling us what is going to bring about the most health-filled outcome, the most beneficial gift to ourselves and to others.

So the next time you feel the need for a little instant gratification, remember that some of the greatest gifts we can give and receive are those moments when we act now, think later.

Spontaneous Healing

I am a planner. I like to organize, have a schedule, and follow along with life in a timely fashion. I have wall calendars, wallet calendars, even phone and email calendars. But I discovered how unexpected health often reveals itself in spontaneity.

There are numerous ways that health plays out when we have no set plans: being spontaneous allows for unexpected adventures to occur, spontaneity allows us to dabble in creative freedom, and being plan-less gives us permission to let ourselves off our own regimented "hooks." But the unexpected health that you won't find penciled in any calendar is that being spontaneous can make you feel like a kid again... And remembering what our lives are like without all of our own headaches is healthy.

On a weekend in San Francisco, I enjoyed having a kid-like day. I tromped around the city with good friends, in great weather, surrounded by lots of activities and opportunities. I have to admit, I did know who I was going with and had an idea of a group meeting spot, but other than that, the day and night were ours to create. There is so much freedom in allowing life to unfold. It is truly amazing what unravels when we let go of the reins.

Our lives are very scheduled, and that is not a bad thing. I think we do better in life when we have some order to our day. But once in a while, it is essential to remember what life was like when we were kids, at least for many of us. Most kids do not have to carry the weight of the world on their shoulders. They are free to explore, to create, to express. We as adults need those spontaneous moments in our lives. We need reminders of the joy that arises when we let go of control.

So the next time you are planning a weekend, don't. Make a reservation or two but leave everything else to opportunity. You may be surprised by how healthy an unplanned adventure can be.

A Call for Health

Life has a funny way of forcing us to speak our truth. We can avoid the conversations as much as we like but truth always prevails. And the more serious the situation, the more our mouth filters come off and our truth-telling sets in. These are the times when we tend to avoid the political correctness, the sparing of feelings, and the holding of our tongues. Because of these truthful and healthy opportunities, I find that unexpected health can infiltrate us with wake-up calls.

Now let me be clear, I am not talking about calls we get in the middle of the night from friends who think we should be joining in their festivities. I am talking about those moments when we are either receiving or giving a hit-you-over-the-head-with-truth reality check on life as we know it. Of course, we all know there are obvious health benefits to wake-up calls. These attention-grabbers give us a new perspective on life to consider, wake-up calls grant us (or others) another chance, an opportunity to re-write our current situation, and being "awakened" (as I've said before) forces us to snap out of whatever daze we are in and pay attention to what life is telling us. But the unexpected health that I am reminded about is that wake-up calls create honesty, and being honest with ourselves and our loved ones is healthy.

I have been given a few wake-up calls in my years of living. My wake-up calls have not always been the result of catastrophic events. In fact, most of them have not been due to tragedy (thankfully). But I have been the recipient of many conversations questioning where I might be going or not going, and what I might be doing or not doing. I have also been the giver of a few wake-up calls. I have had to have those hard conversations with family, with friends, and often the pre-discussion feelings of fear can be tongue-paralyzers. What if they take what I'm saying the wrong way? What if they get mad at me? What if they no longer want to be in my life?

But what I have found is that wake-up calls are perfect opportunities for honest insight and observations. Wake-up calls, whether you are being given one or giving one, remind us that people care. When someone gets angry, sad, upset, or just fed up, and dishes out a little insight, it is often because they love and care about us. If they didn't, why would they waste their breath talking about it? They wouldn't.

I find that those who have been at the receiving end of a Jaime wake-up call are those whom I really love. The people that voice the most concern or even anger when they see those around them acting less than healthy are the same people who would be by your side if a true catastrophic wake-up call was to come into your life.

So the next time you feel bombarded with some hard-hitting information from a loved one, consider their position. Remember that from where they stand, they see someone they love living a life that may be less than their potential. And if you are considering giving that long overdue wake-up call, do it. If we speak our truth in love, with love, love is the only call we are making.

Timekeepers of Health

Although this revelation of health would not be possible without numbers, the almighty numeral is not my helpful tidbit of insight. Because I discovered the unexpected health in calendars.

I'm sure you could give me a list of healthiness scribbled in the boxed-in days of a calendar: calendars help organize our lives (healthy: check), visual reminders allow us to look forward to upcoming events (healthy: check), and of course, a calendar helps us immensely health-promoting, overextended individuals keep our days (or hours, minutes, lunch breaks) on task (healthy: check). But the unexpected health in calendars is that these little squares of days promote community support, and receiving community support is healthy.

Calendars help friends and loved ones plan vacations. Calendars help us count down the days until graduation, a wedding, a holiday, the birth of a baby. Calendars can also be the timekeepers for scary events. People pencil in their day of surgery, their day for making big decisions, for life choices and changes. You tend to find these dates housed right alongside the anniversaries, doctor's appointments, and birthdays. But the blessing of calendars is that if you share these dates, these times, and these events, you give your network of support the opportunity to gather around you, to rally for your health and happiness.

One time, I was surprised as my friends and family rallied together to schedule themselves to prepare food for someone needing some extra TLC on their dinner plate. That's what communities do for each other. When we share our calendar days, those times we want and need extra love and support, don't be surprised if the humanity of others shows up to pencil themselves in too.

So the next time you circle an important date on your own calendar, remember to leave a little extra room for others to join in. Whether it be an exciting day or an upcoming trying time, you may be healthfully surprised by the support you receive. So, mark it on your calendar, and then make it public.

This Just In: Health Being Discovered in the Unknown

Didn't we all want to be rich and famous at some point during our growing up years? Haven't we all had those daydreams of being endlessly wealthy, wildly successful, and insanely well known? Maybe some still long for these aspirations. In my earlier years, I wanted to be anything from a big-time New York magazine writer (step aside, Carrie Bradshaw!), to a professional volleyball player, to a highly paid sales rep. Newsflash: sales is not my strength! But as I read the saddening headlines exploiting the private lives of very public people, I realized how unexpectedly healthy it is to be totally unknown.

Being rich and famous comes with some pretty incredible perks: you can afford any and every variety of luxurious pampering available, you can enjoy getaways to exotic places whenever you choose, you have access to the most high-quality foods, have them bought and prepared for you, and you can then afford to pay someone to clean up the kitchen mess that you didn't even make. But the unexpected health in being an unknown is that you can expose what you choose to expose… And having choices in your personal affairs is healthy.

Online I see headline after headline of juicy famous people gossip, heartaches and headaches. It's not to say that we common folk avoid these types of situations, but when hard times happen, we get to choose who knows our business and who we share our heartache with, instead of being smeared on the cover of People. We lower-tax-bracket individuals financially make less but can emotionally gain so much more... Mainly, our privacy. We are awarded the luxury of privacy, intimacy, and normalcy.

So the next time you feel you are not keeping up with the Joneses, remember that the Jones family may look good on paper, but chances are, their lives are riddled with public humiliation, exploitation, and scrutiny. Consider your quaint little life a comfortable, private, and healthy place to be.

Moisture-Rich Health

I had acne as a teen. I can't remember how bad it was, but I do remember that I did not like it. In fact, I hated it! I used to get so jealous when I would see other kids my age who had baby soft skin. And of course, I tried everything. I used Retin-A, had peels that nearly fried my face off (I hope my mom got her money back for that one!), and eventually resorted to the now extremely popular ProActiv (before Jessica Simpson came on board). But after layers of skin were peeled off and countless towels were stained from ProActiv (anything that bleaches out fabrics has to be too harsh for your skin!), nothing seemed to work... That is, until I started on a much larger-scaled journey of whole health, health that digs in to find out the root cause of dis-ease and discomfort. I switched from harsh chemicals to skin food... Yes, the products I use could literally be consumed. And why shouldn't our skincare be food? The skin is the largest organ in our body, so it makes sense to feed our body's largest organ with the most organic, whole, and healthy products possible, right?! Well, discovering the essential nutrients in skin food, and more importantly, meeting an amazing skin healer along the way, has taught me that unexpected health exfoliates our lives with acne.

Yes, you read that correctly. I am going to somehow manage to prove that there is health in acne. Acne is (literally!) a surface-level indicator. When our faces are blemish-laden, it is an indicator that something is awry, and receiving visual clues to unhealthiness in our lives is healthy.

Acne reveals our imbalances: a hormonal imbalance, a nutritional imbalance, even a life imbalance. We can easily get clogged with stressors in our life, which prevent us from paying attention. So, breakouts are actually wake-up calls for areas we need to pay attention to. In a way, a breakout is actually a breakthrough. Imperfections break through our skin, revealing to us that change in our current situation is necessary. We, in some way, need to *break out* of whatever predicament we might be in.

I have always worn my stress on my face. When I have too much on my plate and do not listen to my inner voice, my skin will find its own version of a bullhorn to yell into... Hello breakout! So now, when my skin is feeling less than optimal, I skip the trip to the pharmacy for blemish-be-gone cream, and instead partake in the "What's going on in your world that you're trying to ignore, Jaime?" conversation that I have needed to have for a while.

So the next time you look in the mirror and wonder why in your thirties, forties, or fifties (or sixties and seventies) you are still having breakouts, consider your little imperfections a sign that something deeper, something below the epidermis, is going on. Look for the breakthrough with your next breakout.

A Healthy Resemblance

The first day of spring is a time of new growth, new beginnings, fresh flowers, and fresh perspectives. One spring equinox, I decided to go for an extra-long hike out in nature with my pooch Lucca, in a perfect location for seeing and experiencing all that a spring day should look like. Green grass, rolling hills, poppies peppering the hillside with a radiant orange hue that literally *pops* up from the ground. Loads of people and their bikes, their children and of course, their dogs, were out on this day of Equinox. As I hiked, I made a conscious effort to talk to as many passersby as I could. Sometimes it was a simple, "Good morning!" Other times, I would stop and let Lucca and another dog chase each other while I had a conversation with the dog's human friend. I'm not typically a bragging sort of dog owner, but I have to admit, everyone who saw Lucca that day made a comment about how cute she was, how happy she seemed to be, and how friendly she was. Now, for those of you who know Lucca, "friendly" may not be the adjective you would have chosen. While she adores those she feels comfortable with, she can be a little, let's say, stand-offish toward those she doesn't know. But out in our open space, she really does turn into a more adapted animal. But this post is not a play-by-play about that morning with my dog. I do have some unexpected health to share and Lucca is a part of my revelation. As others constantly reminded me about my adorable dog, I discovered the unexpected health in resemblances.

Now before I go on, I will admit that this book has forced me to come clean with my readers. I have had to shelve my pride and my privacy at times in order for my insights to make sense. So, here it goes...

I bought Lucca (for twelve dollars I might add—best twelve dollars I ever spent!) because she was a dead-on lookalike of another dog that was once in my life, my ex's family dog. When I saw Lucca's picture, I thought that she looked just like the dog I grew to love during my relationship. More disclosure: I also thought I wanted the lifestyle, the family name, even the location that this pup lived. I thought I wanted to be surrounded by the world she dwelled in. So to me, Lucca was a step toward getting back to the place I had been a few years earlier, to a relationship I thought I wanted to return to.

But the irony, and more importantly, the health that I discovered while I looked at my dog, is how overwhelmingly consumed I was by the love I have for my life, my location, and my dog. I may have initially bought Lucca based on my recollection of a memory, a time in the past, a relationship of the past, but it doesn't matter. When I finally found a picture of my ex's dog, I realized that Lucca actually doesn't really look like her at all. My dog (not my ex's) has helped me grow, expand, and experience a substantial amount of health. She continually surprises me in unexpected ways by the many metaphors she represents in my life: where I've been, where I am, where I'm going.

So the next time you feel that heart-tug need to do something based on a resemblance of someone or some time, remember my story. Remember that you never know how a resemblance to one thing, one person, one experience, can actually become a more expansive channel for you to experience optimal and continual health.

Head Full of Health

I pride myself on not getting sick, not having headaches, and feeling pretty healthy overall, so at one point, I gave away my western medicine—headache, cold, and sinus remedies—and decided I would stock my shelves with more holistic, more homeopathic healing agents. I replaced Advil with tea tree oil, Pepto Bismol with peppermint tea and lavender oil, and Benadryl with a Neti pot (for those of you have never used a Neti pot, you're in for a real treat!).

But nonetheless, no matter how lovely my healing remedies may be, I still hate being sick, so you can imagine my frustration when I found myself having a throbbing headache for an entire weekend. Because of this head pounding annoyance, I felt compelled to discover the unexpected health in a headache. Here is my attempt at some helpful insight...

Headaches literally force me to stay home, physically and mentally. When I have a vision-blurring kind of headache, I have no other choice but to clear my mind. Headaches shove out any available space in my head, and for me, that is a healthy necessity at times. My mind can go from zero to sixty miles per hour in no time at all, but headaches act as that emergency brake that I need to remind myself to slow down, take it easy, and stop thinking once in a while. Having these mental and physical e-brakes installed in ourselves is healthy.

I spent most of that time in my house, watching movies, something I rarely do. After teaching my nutrition class, I ran a few errands, but then I immediately went back to the couch to watch my third chick flick of the weekend.

It's hard to give ourselves permission to chill out. Our society does not look fondly on couch potatoes. To be honest, I don't either. But sometimes, when our worlds become too busy and our minds become too cluttered, a little R&R is the best remedy. Unfortunately for most of us, it takes an illness like a headache to give us permission to relax, to unwind, to just be.

So the next time you feel yourself getting worn down, overly tired, or just plain sick, give yourself permission to recuperate, rejuvenate, and recharge. Consider your next headache, stomachache, backache, neckache, or toothache a reminder that if we overdo it in life, we can only go so long until our bodies put on the brakes. Remember that if you don't take care of yourself, how can you possibly have anything to share with the world?

Lost and Found

I would consider myself an organized person. Actually, I am annoyingly organized. I feel some self-disclosure coming on: I line cans up in a cabinet so they all face the same way. I absolutely hate hand-written tabs on folders (yes, I own a label maker). My computer desktop is clutter-free, easy to navigate and all folders are well labeled. But despite my obsessiveness with organization, I discovered that there is *some* (and I do emphasize *some*) unexpected health to be found when you lose something.

I am referring to the piece of paper, the folder, or the shopping list that you just know you've seen but for the life of you, you cannot find it! You know what I'm talking about: you can visually see what the missing object looks like ("It's this long sheet of lined paper that has a cow on the top that says, 'Mooove It or Lose It' underneath the udders"—something like that). You can remember picking it up, setting it down. You can recall the day you had it, who you were with, what you were wearing, and where you were going. But for some strange reason, you have *no idea* where the darned thing is. That happened to me one day. In my compulsive organization, I had still managed to lose something.

As I was rifling through my office, which was then desk-free (I blamed that fact for my lost paperwork!), I discovered some tidbits of information that I had forgotten I owned. A few years earlier, I started collecting sayings that I loved. As you can imagine, because of my love affair with words, I found pages and pages of inspirational quotes, thought-provoking sayings, and life-changing challenges. These had been tucked away (neatly, of course), so while I was on a paper hunt, I re-discovered the inspiration I had been collecting... And unexpectedly discovering inspiration is healthy.

When we lose things, we are forced to look. We see our house, our office, our car, even our life, with a different lens. When life is going normally, it is easy to overlook those healthy reminders that are often right in front of our noses. When something is taken away, temporarily misplaced, or permanently removed, we cannot help but see life in a different light. It commonly happens that when I lose something, I discover something more. I might have lost a piece of paper that day, but I found some healthy insights that I obviously needed to read.

So the next time you lose a document, a to-do list, or an important piece of paper, start looking. But open your eyes a little wider, expand your heart a little wider, and search for something more. You may never find your missing work, but I guarantee you will find a reminder, a memento, or an inspiration that you just may need that day.

Single Dose of Health

Have I mentioned how much I love spring? On a very warm, sunny, spring day, Lucca and I went for a run. My day had been pretty hectic, so I needed to get a little more oxygen into my lungs and even more information out of my mind. During my run, I tried to notice the nature that surrounded me. I saw the coyote that Lucca desperately wanted to play with (but thankfully didn't!). I came up close and personal to a herd of cows. But toward the end of my nature jaunt, I discovered a piece of unexpected health that caught my attention: the health we discover, unexpectedly, from being singled out.

Having someone single you out can be horrifying. That spotlight of embarrassment can shine right on us when we get pointed out of a crowd, are singled out in a group, or noticed for some particular reason. And oftentimes, being singled out is associated with a negative event. As kids, did you ever get called out in class for being disruptive, wrong, or out of line? Not me! (Obviously, that is a joke...)

Anyway, the unexpected health we retain from being the subject of singled-outness (I think I just made up a word) is that when we are positioned away from the crowd, we have the ability to reveal our one-of-a-kind selves... And showcasing our unique specialness to the world is healthy.

Let's get back on track… I started this post about my run. At the very end of my run, I noticed one lone poppy alongside a hill of weeds, brownish grass, and rocks. Although most of our neighborhood open space is lush and green right now, this particular location is blah and brown. But not that day. Well, at least, I didn't notice it until then. This one orange flowering beauty had pronounced itself among a setting of nothing eye-catching or particularly unique. But the poppy caught my attention.

It is easy to blur into the landscape of life, of our society, our culture. It takes guts to be brave, to stand out in a crowd, to be singled out. Now of course, I am not promoting we all act out in order to be singled out… Of course not! But I do encourage each and every one of us to highlight our own uniqueness. Those in our history books are not there because they played it safe and never colored outside the lines of life. In fact, just the opposite. People that make history do so because they are not afraid of being singled out, called out, or even cast out.

So the next time you feel the urge to take a stand, be bold! Stand out! You just never know what kind of history you might be making.

Shopping for Health

I used to be a big-time shopper. I was never a high-end buyer. I was the type who may not spend five hundred dollars on one pair of Manolo Blahniks but would have thirty pairs of shoes that equaled the same amount of money. In my mind, I was justified because I was getting more bang for my buck. In other words, I was an advertiser's ideal customer!

As I have tried to clear the clutter out of my life (literally and figuratively!), I have eased up on my frivolous spending. But every now and again, I like a nice new outfit, a cute pair of shoes, or a new sun dress. And because of a recent shopping experience, I discovered the unexpected health one can find hanging on the sale rack while shopping!

I'm sure at this point, every woman reading this just got really excited. Yes, there *is* health to be had in the Nordstrom, Macy's, and Target near you! But in my experience, what you take off the hanger is not nearly as important or as healthy as what you put on the minds of store employees.

Let me explain: I bought a pair of jeans one time. Because I am not the tallest woman in the world, I needed to get them shortened. So I put them on, had them pinned, and then handed them off to the lady who does the alterations. We walked to the counter, rang up my items, and away I went. A week or so later, I picked them up and now have the cutest, gemstone-pocketed jeans around! Later on, I decided I needed to return one of the items that I just didn't like. But before I went, I checked my mail and saw that my store's credit card statement was in my mailbox. So, I opened it and looked at the total... Surprisingly low! What I noticed was that I hadn't been charged for my jeans—quite a dilemma. Do I plead not guilty and enjoy a free pair of jeans? Not my mistake, right? Isn't that a healthy little freebie?

Well, I walked in, returned my unwanted item, and then paused... The unexpected health in shopping is that even when we are buying objects for ourselves, indulging in our desires, we can still show healthy behaviors for a higher good... And promoting good in any and every opportunity is healthy. Shifting from a "me" mentality to a "we" way of living and being begins the much-needed paradigm shift in our world, a shift toward seeking the goodness for all instead of the benefit of self.

So the next time you have an opportunity to show unexpectedly positive behavior, do not let this opportunity pass you by. Even if it costs you more money or if it inconveniences you a little, remember that our world cannot change if it doesn't start with just one person... Let that one person be you. That day, I walked to the jeans section, grabbed the same pair of jewel-pocketed jeans I had at home, took them to the counter, paid for them, and walked out empty handed, but full of integrity.

The Dawn of Health

I am a neat freak. I cannot leave the house without making my bed. I cringe at dishes in the sink, water stains on the mirrors and unfolded decorative towels. After re-reading what I just wrote, it should come as no surprise that my life is, what some might call, a little wound up at times. But as I came home to a messy kitchen (a rarity in this house!), I thought, as I scrubbed pans, wooden spoons, and bowls of all sizes, how unexpected health suds up in our life while doing dishes.

The chore that sends most people into a tizzy is actually filled to the brim with health. Now of course, there are obvious health benefits to doing the dishes: antibacterial dishwashing liquid comes to mind. Obviously, removing the germs from your dishware is healthy. But the unexpected health that can never be washed away with the leftovers is that washing dishes means that you dirtied dishes. Dirty dishes mean that you cooked something. Hopefully, you cooked something healthy for yourself and maybe even someone else... And nourishing your body with healthy foods is healthy.

Okay, so not everyone who dirties up a kitchen is cooking healthy foods. Of course not. But the more often you choose not to eat the processed, packaged, frozen, pre-made, and ready-to-be-eaten-in-two-minutes microwave meals, the greater the likelihood you will cook. And I have found that if you cook, you may just squeeze in a few leafy green goodies into the stir fry, salad bowl or chicken dish. But you can't create these culinary concoctions without dirtying up a few dishes.

I had made a mess the day before. I had a pile of dishes in the sink and on the counter the following morning. But I didn't wake up feeling agitated by the mess I had made. I was bubbled over with happiness from the healthy meal I had prepared for myself, along with a little savory soup I made for a friend. Although I created dirty dishes, I also encouraged clean eating.

It is easy to get busy. Our lives are hurried, so it makes sense to grab the quick, ready-made meals in our freezers. But, when we take the time to nourish ourselves with "live" food (not food that dwells in a box), we are promoting life and health in ourselves.

So the next time you debate whether to pull out the microwave meal or dig through your fridge's crisper drawer, choose to dirty up your dishes and cook yourself a meal. You may have more of a mess in the kitchen, but you'll definitely have *less* of a mess in your belly.

Becoming the Patient

I had been trying to create my home office for months when I finally found the perfect desk to accent my vibrant turquoise walls. Throughout the course of my research, I saw tons of desks: wooden desks, modern desks, L-shaped desks (which is what I wanted), roll-top desks, student desks... I never knew there could be so many varieties of desks! But I was particular about what I wanted: an L-shaped glass top, rounded corners (feng shui says to eliminate sharp edges on furniture), and a dark wood (preferably cherry).

The desk I initially ordered had two of the three requirements, and I had to assemble it, which I wouldn't say I like doing. My mindset was, "Well, two of my requirements is better than nothing... Maybe this is the best I can get." Not so. This brings me to the unexpected health insight: the amazingly healthy result one can experience in patience.

Now, as I have disclosed before, patience is not one of my virtues. I have to work hard to wait. But as I sat at my new desk, overlooking my patio and feeling the cool breeze flowing through the room, I experienced the fantastic reward that being patient grants us.

It is so easy to be impatient, and unfortunately, we live in a society where we wait for nothing. We have overnight delivery, online shopping, digital cameras, ten-day escrow options. The times of saving, waiting, and wondering are of the past. But sometimes (actually, most of the time), waiting and holding out for what we desire is the most gratifying reward we can give ourselves.

So the next time you are wavering on whether to take the plunge on something that isn't exactly what you're looking for, hold out! When we practice patience and wait for what we really want, the reward is so much greater.

Talking Shoes

It's easy to tell people what they want to hear. I have never found conformity to be a challenge. And I'm sure both humans and salmon would agree that it is much easier to go with the flow instead of trying to swim upstream in life. But while cruising around my house doing some organizing (my favorite pastime), I discovered the unexpected health of walking.

Now at this point, you might be wondering what salmon spawning has to do with health and walking. Well, to be honest, it doesn't. But, just as these omega-3-packed fish must swim against the flow every year, unexpected health is readily available when we stand for what we believe, when we *walk* our talk.

Physically walking is healthy, of course. There is no need to review the many health benefits of moving our little legs about. But walking our talk is also an extremely healthy practice because when we stand up for what we believe, we embody the words that we speak by creating cohesion with our actions.

Anyone can speak a bunch of gibberish. Telling others what they want to hear while acting another way is easy. But when we choose to match our words with our actions, when we walk our talk, that takes courage... And being courageous in life is healthy.

I try my best to live how I believe, to create words in form. If what I say does not match how I act, then I am a fraud. Those who inspire others, who make an imprint in our lives, are not those who say one thing and do another. It's not that we will ever be perfect all the time or that our words and actions will always match up. We are human, and part of our humanness is making mistakes, acting with less integrity than we know we possess. But we create health for ourselves and others by standing by our beliefs and refusing to allow unjust behavior to prevail.

So the next time you are faced with an idea or an action that you do not agree with, put on your integrity shoes and walk! Do not be afraid of rocking the boat... In life, there is often no change without a few waves.

Not Your Typical Health Store

I have to admit, I like grocery shopping. Well, let me rephrase: I like grocery shopping at health food stores. Unfortunately, these stores aren't nearly as reasonable as your typical Grocery Outlet, WinCo Foods, or Food 4 Less. But I will tell you, they are way more fun. There are always yummy goodies to try (which may be why you'll spend eight dollars for a block of cheese that you could get for four dollars at Safeway), lots of funky foods to buy (kale crisps anyone?), and there is never a shortage of fruits and vegetables that you have never heard of before. But while shopping at the typically boring chain grocery store down the street, I found some unexpected health in shopping carts!

Now, you might be asking yourself, "How in the world can shopping carts be healthy? Don't they provide sanitizer wipes near shopping carts because they are so unhealthy?" Well, my soapbox discussion on how we are over sanitized is a whole other issue that I will not delve into right now. Of course, shopping carts can house all sorts of health-filled items: fruits, veggies, whole grains, wine! But the unexpected health that we push around with shopping carts is that when you check out of the grocery store and walk out into the parking lot, you have this incredible opportunity to let go. Try it: place one foot on the lower rack, give your-self a little push, raise your other foot onto that same rack, hold on, and sail your way to your car! Let's be honest, who doesn't enjoy a little ride on the back of a shopping cart?

While doing the very mundane activity of grocery shopping, I ended my outing with a little joyride. I felt, if even just for a minute or so, like a kid without a care or responsibility in the world. I placed my adults-don't-do-this ego in my metal cart and away I went… And being able to let go of our endless adultness once in a while is healthy.

Life can be so serious sometimes. Once we get out of school, we are expected to act a certain way, to maintain composure, to be cool and collected. Well guess what? Sometimes we need to remind our uber-responsible selves that life is too short to take every moment so seriously.

So the next time you have the daunting task of after-work grocery shopping, when the lines are longer and people's fuses are shorter, create a little fun, a little health, with your experience. Hop on, hold on, and take a spin with your shopping cart. You are never too old to have a little childish fun.

Health Expectations

I expect a lot from myself and hold myself to a very high standard. This mentality creates both health and disharmony in my life.

The healthy aspect of my high expectations is that I get tasks done effectively, professionally, and on time. People know they can rely on me because I am responsible and keep my word. However, this elevated expectation I place on myself can also lead to burnout because if I know I can do something, I am determined to do it *myself*. One day, however, amid my self-expectations as well as the expectations I put on my surroundings, I discovered some unexpected large-scale health in high expectations!

Let me explain: I had been trying to rent this abnormally large, somewhat unique office space for quite a few months. When the previous tenant moved out, I walked in and immediately envisioned a specific type of business that would be perfect for the space: a movement and healing center. We opened up the room to create one large spacious area, put hardwood floors in, and painted the walls a neutral but warm color. I could see the yoga mats rolled up in a basket in the corner. I imagined quiet music, mindful movement, and awareness education. I know it sounds weird, but that's what I saw. I even posted a Craigslist ad describing my vision, stating something like, "This space is perfect for a yoga and/or pilates studio." Really, that's what it said.

Well one afternoon, I received a phone call from an inquirer. They had not even seen the Craigslist blurb, which expressed my high hopes for the space. Instead, they saw our sign dangling from the roof. Fast forward to this afternoon and what you will find is a completed lease application for the prospective tenant. There it was, right in front of me! It is a healthy practice to have high expectations! The prospective tenant's occupation was exactly aligned with the intention that I put out into the world and onto my Craigslist account.

As much as I can burn myself out with my unrealistic expectations, the unexpected health I find might be worth it. When we refuse to waiver, when we set the bar a little higher than expected, we are often pleasantly (and unexpectedly) surprised by the outcome. On that day, I visually saw what happens when we keep our eye on the ball and expect nothing less than what is optimally healthy for the greater good... And helping create health for more than ourselves is healthy.

So the next time you find yourself settling into comfort, I challenge you to take it to the next level. I propose you set the bar a little higher, set your expectations slightly above, and just see what happens. You might find yourself burned out... or you might find your passion, your happiness, your health, burning from the inside out.

Changing Our View of Health

You've heard the old adage, "A penny saved is a penny earned," right? Or, "A penny for your your thoughts." Or the now highly outdated, "Here's a quarter, call someone who cares."

Obviously, that last saying is archaic. Do you ever actually even *see* payphones anymore? That is beside the point. What I am getting at is that coins are essential, yet oftentimes annoyances, in our life... Well, at least they are in mine. Excess change weighs down my wallet, spills in my car, and tumbles around in my wash. And, of course, coins are found in all sorts of strange and unclean places, making coins a questionably unhealthy object. But one day, I discovered unexpected health in, you guessed it, loose change.

That morning, I met my good friend for a quick cup of coffee (you've already heard me rhapsodize on the benefits of coffee!). We grabbed our drinks and sat outside to catch up for just a few minutes. All of a sudden, who do we see barreling down the street in their Barbie-sized mode of transportation? The meter person! We got up and began scurrying to our cars to check our meter, because let's face it, a nice cup of coffee catch-up with a good friend can easily be ruined by a little white envelope resting in your windshield wiper. Just as we arrived at my car (which had run out of time), a complete stranger saw the meter person giving tickets, and immediately fed my meter. Someone who had no idea whose car it was took some of his spare change and *spared* me an expensive parking ticket.

Loose change allows us to unexpectedly create happiness in another's day... And bringing about happiness is not only healthy, it is contagious.

When you have a little extra change in your pocket, your purse, or your piggy bank, think of all the ways you can pay it forward: you could pleasantly surprise others by randomly feeding their meters when it is out of time. One more quarter might allow a homeless person to buy that sandwich that was just above their budget. And a few more coins might just fund an orphanage in another country or an outreach program on our own soil. As much as spare change may weigh down your personal belongings, think about how much pain, suffering, and sadness could be lifted for another with that same number of coins.

So the next time you feel your spare change weighing you down, find a small bag or coin purse and keep it: keep it in your car, in your purse, or in your briefcase, and when you see an opportunity to pay it forward, do it. Feed a meter. Buy a lunch. Donate. You just never know the pain you may be sparing by giving away a few extra coins. And to the gentleman who fed my meter today, thank you. I will do my part and pay it forward to someone else.

Seated at the Right Hand of Health

After I found my perfect desk, I became obsessed with my new home office. I loved it: my feng shui–approved L-shaped desk, my view to the outside world, and the topic of this particular unexpected health insight is my comfy office chair. Yes, health is seated on the cushion of a good old-fashioned swiveling office chair.

Now, there are many healthy aspects of an office chair: you've got a place to rest your rump during the work day. Office chairs often come equipped with adjustable heights, arm rests, even uprightness. But the unexpected health in office chairs is that the simple swiveling mechanism that sets a desk chair apart from the rest allows us to change perspectives by literally changing our position... And having a perspective change is healthy.

Think about it: you can be faced with one problem, one task, one horribly annoying individual... all facing one direction. But, with a slight abdominal movement or push with your hand, you can literally and physically face something entirely different. Oftentimes when we feel frustrated or stuck in a specific situation, we find not-so-healthy coping mechanisms: we eat, we gulp down a large amount of caffeine, we bite our fingernails, we email our friend to gripe and complain. But really, sometimes all we need to do is turn our chair and our environment toward something different, which means our lookout can change our outlook.

Sometimes we need to change directions, change positions, and change perspectives. Our vision in life can get rather blurry when we over-focus on life's ups and downs.

So the next time you are troubled at work, consider a turnaround of thought with the turn of your chair. We are equipped with all sorts of healthy and helpful tools for living in this life... We just need to remember to look for them. And sometimes, just sometimes, we are seated on top of them.

Burning with Health

We all have ways of coping with stress. As I have self-disclosed many times already, I can be a bit wound up at times, so it is imperative that I have a variety of stress-relieving practices. Did you all know that April is Stress Awareness Month? I'd say that's pretty perfect since it is also tax time (I'm sure there are no coincidences there!).

So one April, I tried to focus on how I could eliminate stress from my life and since that is nearly impossible, I focused more clearly on how to relieve my stress.

Without thinking too hard, I discovered a powerful stress-reducing, unexpected health insight from burning incense.

I have always had a therapeutic relationship with incense, especially Nag Champa. I have burned many different types of incense, but Nag Champa is definitely my favorite. And one day, after coming home from a less-than-stress-free afternoon, I realized that burning incense actually relieves my stress... And finding *any* sort of stress-relieving self-care practice is healthy.

What's interesting about my unexpected health discovery is that I didn't know that incense was healthy until I took in the aroma. So, of course, as soon as I got home, I immediately went and put incense in *both* incense holders and smoked out the house with the aroma of this sweet Middle Eastern scent. But once I sat down to write, I noticed that I began feeling more peaceful. As the aroma filled the room, my mind cleared, my body relaxed, and my blood pressure undoubtedly dropped.

This stress-alleviating stick prompted me to look up what Nag Champa is made of (don't get me started on the unexpected health in research!). It turns out that Nag Champa contains a large concentration of sandalwood. And sandalwood, in alternative medicine, is believed to bring one closer to the "Divine"—or God, Buddha, whatever your belief may be. Sandalwood is also considered a remedy for anxiety. Who knew?!

Sometimes it seems that we mindlessly do things: take a walk, go out to dinner, call a friend, burn fragrant aromas into the air. But I find that for every day-to-day activity, there is usually something deeper at work. For example, I have burned more incense in the past few months than I have in a very long time. When I look back, I can see that I have allowed my life to become rather stressful, which in turn, has drawn me toward Nag Champa incense, my very own stress-relieving aid.

So the next time you feel stress in your life, pay attention to the objects, people, and surroundings you are drawn to. I bet there is no coincidence that when times get tough, you will unconsciously (or consciously) gravitate toward ease in your day, your mind, your life. Our bodies are not meant for excess stress. So when we get in those places of anxiousness, our bodies will find ways back to homeostasis… maybe one incense stick at a time.

Filing a Health Claim

I was born on April 15, also known as tax day... That's not a day I would like to be born on. It's hard to be born on one of the most dreaded days of the year. Well, as this capital-T Time quickly approached, I had countless questions (both asked of me as well as those I've asked), created numerous reports, and rummaged through piles of the previous year's files. Finally, shuffled in with all of the tax prep paperwork, I have found some unexpected health in (yes, I'm going to say it) taxes!

Having had three different lengthy conversations with the accountant about my taxes, it was difficult to think of the apparent health benefits of taxes. I'm not sure if there are known health advantages to the tax season. It does seem correlated with other "seasons" in our lives: cold, allergy, and flu season come to mind—much like tax season, not an enjoyable time in our lives! But the less-than-obvious, unexpected ways that taxes are healthy, show up not on our 1099s and W2s. Instead, they show up in our mindsets.

Taxes offer us (like other opportunities in our lives) a chance at a clean slate... And being able to start fresh is healthy. Whatever happened in the previous year is put to rest when we mail in our forms to the IRS. That fiscal year is over, no matter how financially good or bad it was. If the previous year was a little rough, it is over. We are in a new year, full of new possibilities and experiences. If the previous year was unimaginably fantastic, then you will always have a standard by which to measure greatness. We will not always have horribly devastating or blissfully happy years. Such is life. But, when we file our taxes, we are given a blank canvas on which to create our upcoming year, our life, and of course, our health.

So the next time April 15 approaches, consider it a day not to dread but to embrace. File your return but save an extra stamp. Along with your paperwork, postmark your unwanted experiences of the previous year, and mentally mail those as well. And if you are one of those serial extension filers, consider this year your last... Because the longer you extend your past, the longer it will take you to live in the now and prepare for the future.

Hitting the Health Notes

I am no Lady Gaga. I may sing in the shower and belt out a tune in my car (while driving with the sunroof open, of course), but there are no record deals coming my way.

However, while watching a group of singers on TV and singing to my own tune most days, I perked up my ears and listened to some unexpected health that hits the health note in singing.

Now, singing has all sorts of physical health benefits: the vibration that travels through your body when you sing acts as an internal massage, calming and soothing our organs. Hitting a big note forces us to practice diaphragmatic breathing, also healthy. And belting out a happy tune can lift our spirits. But the unexpected health benefit of singing is that when you take the time to memorize the lyrics, mimic the melody, and squawk out the tune, you are expressing your emotions... And freeing your innermost thoughts into form is healthy.

Ever wonder why you hit the "Repeat" button with your favorite song? Find it strange that you gravitate toward certain songs more than others? Sometimes we love a song because of the catchy tune, but we often favor a song because of its lyrics. When we consciously or unconsciously feel a certain way, songs give us the avenue, the permission, to express it in words. For example, on days I feel sad, I have found that I tend to belt out, hit "Repeat," and belt out again a song that speaks to my feelings. On the other hand, days when I feel happy and energetic, I have the toe-tapping need to use my pipes for a lively beat.

It's hard to be open with our feelings sometimes. Some say that men are the ones who have trouble tapping into their deeper selves, but as a woman, I can be reserved with my emotions as well. So when I need a filter for my feelings, an outlet for a healthy expression, singing allows me that opportunity.

So the next time you hear a song and get lost in the lyrics and mesmerized by the melody, remember the song that tugs at your heart is a compilation of words to pay attention to.

Soaring Toward Health

Traveling by plane can be quite an ordeal. Before board-ing, you must park your car, take a shuttle to the terminal, unload your luggage, walk to the check-in counter, and shuffle through your wallet looking for confirmations, IDs, and boarding passes. Then it's off to security. Stand in line. Show your boarding pass and ID again, take off your shoes, coat, vest, jewelry, and belt. Next, you will walk through security, hope you don't get stopped, pull out all the gear you just dumped into the little plastic bin, and away you go looking for your gate. Finally, you spot it, and you arrive at your gate only to wait in more lines to board and nearly knock out passengers with your carry-ons while trying to find a seat. If you have my luck, you are stuck in the middle seat, with both armrests already spoken for. Aah, the love of flying.

But as I sat in the middle chair, feeling the little legs behind me pushing against my seat, my arms plastered to my sides, I was reminded of the unexpected health that soars right alongside me while flying.

Flying is often associated with many unhealthy charac-teristics: the recycled air is the culprit of post-landing colds and flu, flights can be nerve-wracking if you are stuck behind or next to a screaming baby, and flying can invoke an array of fears, phobias and anxieties. But the unexpected health that shares space with the friendly skies is that when we are soaring through the clouds, seeing the Earth from a one-of-a-kind lens, we have the opportunity to be reminded about the beauty that surrounds us... And seeing the good on this Earth is healthy. If we let ourselves, it would be easy to be entangled with the negativity of our surroundings. Our eyes and minds are inundated with all of the horrors going on around us: murdered people, kidnapped children, warfare, hate crimes, racial crimes. But once you are in the air, you are forced to unplug from the world below. Flying allows us to look out our window (or peer over the shoulder of the lucky guy sitting in the window seat) and see the beauty and the good.

It's not that we should be naïve to the tragedies around us. But sometimes, just sometimes, we need to be able to fly away from the bad, the sad, and the discouraging.

So the next time you take a trip on a flight, forget about the annoyance of the check-in counter, the security gate, and the baggage claim. Consider your time in the sky a perfect opportunity to see the beauty that still exists amidst the ugliness... Sometimes we just need to elevate ourselves above to see it more clearly. And if you are lucky enough to get a window seat, do your neighbors a favor (unless they are sleeping) and leave the window shade up. Share the beauty with those around you.

Strangely Healthy

I was in Boulder, Colorado one weekend. Before I begin rattling off my health insights, let me say that Southwest Airlines may very well get its own unexpected health day, because if it had not been for our free Companion Passes, my mom and I would not have been there, enjoying the beauty and majesty of this mountain terrain. But here we were after a two-and-a-half hour plane ride landed us in the Rocky Mountains.

I am a huge planner and that means I did a lot of research before we came. For example, I learned about the popular Pearl Street, a fantastic place for shopping, eating, people watching, and sitting in the sun. As we walked around Boulder, we finally decided to ask the locals what else we should see, which was how I discovered the unexpected health of talking to strangers and turning them into friends.

In our society, we teach our children to never talk to strangers because the results can be horribly unhealthy and tragic. But as we grow, we become better equipped with a sensory gauge that warns us when potentially harmful people are in our path. Because of this awareness, we can be pleasantly enlightened and given some unexpected health tidbits from those unknown to us.

A local recommended we drive to the small mountain town of Nederland, approximately twenty minutes outside of Boulder. So, of course, we did. We arrived in this one-horse town and looked for a local coffee shop, which we found. As we started walking toward the entrance, a young guy invited us inside a house-like structure being constructed. My mom and I both hesitated, and sensing our hesitation, this twenty-something-year-old assured us that it was okay and that he had something worth pulling out our camera for. We walked through the plastic tarps that acted as the door, across the flooring, which was peppered with wood shavings, and through another plastic tarp. Then, all of a sudden, we walked into a large, oval-shaped room that housed the most beautiful, most unique carousel I have ever seen... And here it was, placed at over eight thousand feet in a town with a population of probably less than four hundred.

The story behind this masterpiece is that the young guy's dad had been dreaming, planning, and building this structure for over twenty-five years. We later heard that the visionary behind the Carousel of Happiness had been a Vietnam veteran who, after seeing all of the tragedies and sad, wounded children during the war, decided he would come back to the States and create happiness in children's lives. This creative genius had bought various carousel pieces from an auction in Coney Island, where a fire had destroyed the original carousel. He then hand-carved the animals and refurbished this circular play structure that has been bringing smiles to children's lives for a century.

We can see so much more in life when we talk to strangers. I find that as we open up our hearts to those we do not know, we have an opportunity to gain much insight, and much health.

Our excursion out of our comfort zones and into an unknown construction site led us to a visionary's passion taking form. We heard a story that day. We learned how one man took the tragedies he endured and created good for the masses.

So the next time you are interrupted by a stranger, be open to the possibilities and the story you may be witness to. What's so strange about strangers anyway? Most of the time, they are simply people we have yet to meet. And even more often, these unknown people have amazing stories to share.

Homegrown Health

I am a farmer's market junkie. Yep, I am addicted to experiencing the local flare of a town by perusing the tents of their Saturday, Sunday, or weekday market. But one day, as I walked through Boulder's uber chic and cool market, I discovered the unexpected health that sets up shop on a thoroughfare near you at a farmer's market.

Now, of course, there are many obvious health benefits to a farmer's market: you can pick up fresh, local, often organic fruits, vegetables, oils, nut butters, honey, even wine. In addition, a farmer's market makes for a great outing on a beautiful morning, whether with family, friends, or on your own. And a local market displays the area's foods, allowing a greater understanding of local food sources. But the unexpected health you find under the tent-lined street at a farmer's market is that you are experiencing an individual town's culture. Each local farmer's market shows the beauty of that town, and what each artisan offers.

I fell in love with farmer's markets when I lived in Santa Barbara. The Tuesday night market, which blocked off numerous blocks on the famous State Street, offered a glimpse into the health that Santa Barbara offered: lavender oils, fresh tuberoses (which I never find at other markets), local honey, even local dog treats.

After Santa Barbara, I grew to love Chico, California's Thursday night market, which showcased the uniqueness of this college town: kettle corn, gypsy dancers, fresh herbs, and the most amazing breads. And that day, Boulder's Saturday market reached Santa Barbara and Chico caliber for my farmer's market fix.

Each and every one of us has a special gift to share with the world. Some of our gifts are more easily displayed. Teachers have schools at which to display their work. Doctors are often found showcasing their gifts in a hospital. And those wanting to show others the awe of the skies have airline carriers like Southwest Airlines in which to work with. But local artists are often left to a work-out-of-your-home, do-it-yourself, and barely-mowed-grassroots marketing at local venues in which to display their creative expression to the world. Farmer's markets are often those venues.

So the next time you want to experience artistry at work, take a trip to your local farmer's market. You never know what sort of inspiration and what sort of health insights you may gain. And if you are considering a relocation, make sure you see what unique gift your town has the potential to offer by grabbing your recycled bags and making your way down to the farmer's market. You can learn a lot about a place and its people by the farmer's market. So stop by, gather your fresh fruits and veggies, and take a little stroll under the tents toward health.

The Family Doctor

I am surrounded by my family. Literally, my parents and my brother live within five miles of my house. This makes for very convenient holiday get-togethers, Sunday night dinners, and borrowing pots and pans, crock pots, and baking dishes. But today, as I thought about conversations I had and encounters I watched, I discovered the unexpected health that does not always share the same gene pool with family.

Now, this post is not so much about the health we discover unexpectedly with our nuclear families. There are both health benefits and dis-ease that can frame any old family portrait. Instead, I thought about how healthy it is for us to expand our definitions of family.

I am very fortunate. I have an extremely close relationship with my family. But many do not share in my fortune. I also live close to my family, and many do not have that same luxury either. But, no matter how close or how far you may be from your blood relatives, family can be created anywhere, with anybody... And knowing that you have family in your life, watching your back, is healthy.

I was sitting in the hotel common area in Boulder, writing a health insight. I noticed a group of men playing a friendly game of pool and after a few minutes, one of them came over to say hello. Tex was his name. He had come to Boulder five years earlier, and his company had put him up in this hotel while finishing a job. Five years later, Tex was still staying at that hotel as a permanent resident. I watched as Tex talked to all of the wait staff, the housekeepers, the bartenders. Tex had found his home, his family, at a place—a hotel—commonly used for passers-through, weekend visitors, and business travelers. But Tex created a family in the circumstances that life dealt him.

Not everyone is blessed with family closeness. Not every person is lucky enough to live near their family, and others want to live as far away from their relatives as possible. So, we have an incredible health opportunity to create a family—friends and loved ones who you know you can count on, depend on, and lean on even if our blood types, hair color, and eye colors do not match. Family is more than the last name we are born into. Families are those loved ones who, at the end of the day, you know will be there the next.

So the next time you feel you are far away from your home or emotionally distant from your relatives, remember that family is what you create and nurture. It is the closeness you generate with the people in your life, even if those people are your hotel neighbors in the next room.

Getting Away For Health

After an unexpected weekend getaway to the utopia in Colorado, I came back on California soil. Back to work, responsibility, and schedules. The letdown felt on a Sunday night after a much-awaited weekend is always a bit depressing. But as I unpacked my bags and put away the goodies I purchased, I thought about my weekend and how easy it is to experience unexpected health with a quick weekend getaway.

We all look forward to vacations. A long stint away from it all can be so rejuvenating. Of course, there is an abundance of unexpected health that shares luggage space with a long vacation. But short trips, weekends away, are also Samsonite-stuffed with health. It is much easier to pack up a small bag and head outta dodge for a few days than it is to prepare for an extend-a-stay. A short flight may be close to home location-wise, but the distance away from the pressures of life can be monumental. And being able to get away and unwind from the stressors of life is healthy.

Sometimes we need to remove ourselves from our lives to relax physically. And often, it doesn't matter how far the distance is between home and a getaway. The more responsibilities we have, the harder it seems to get away for a long time period. But even a short three-day mini-vacation can give us that jumpstart we need to re-enter the world.

So the next time you feel the need to get away but can't afford or can't commit to being gone for a week or more, consider the invigoration, the health, from a quick trip. You don't have to travel internationally to find some R&R… It may be in your country, in your state, or even in your zip code.

Public Health Reform

I have a healthy fear of public restrooms. Well, maybe fear is a bit of an exaggeration, but I definitely do not like the multiple-stalled, hope-the-hook-for-your-purse-is-still-intact, and lines-out-the-door annoyance of bathrooms. But, being forced to walk through the large "W" door at a public location made me think about health. Yes, this place of known uncleanliness actually caused thoughts of health to swirl around my head, proving that unexpected health can truly be found in the most peculiar places... even public restrooms!

Now, let me better explain my health claims of public facilities. I am in no way suggesting you allow your one-year-old to crawl around the floors of a public restroom. There are all sorts of unhealthful substances lurking in the cracks of a restroom tile floor. Nor are my health claims related to the motion-detected soap dispensers, faucets, and paper towel dispensers (although they too are a healthy bonus to any restroom). What I discovered to be unexpectedly healthy about a public bathroom is not the fancy equipment but the helpful and healthy insights scribbled on the bathroom stall doors. These little scribbles are inspiring and entertaining and therefore healthy!

I am always fascinated by the things people write on

bathroom stalls. Sometimes their words are full of hate, of hurt, or bizarre pictures of cartoon-like characters. But other times, the words you find sharpied on the back of a door cause an immediate self-reflective wonderment and curiosity. "We often miss what we need to see" were the words of wisdom on my bathroom door. Like I said, self-reflection, no matter where you are, is always a helpful practice.

What makes people feel so inspired (or so vandalism-prone) to write something in a place for the whole world to see? What made that person write that statement? Was it meant for herself? Did she intend someone specific to read it? Maybe she posted it as a reminder for all to read? Whatever the reason, I appreciated the reflective statement (although I do not condone vandalizing any public location, no matter how inspirational your message may be). I couldn't help but smile and wonder how I can better see those things, those people, those experiences that I so easily overlook in my life.

So the next time you find yourself in a public restroom, look for the healthy insights... They could be scribbled on the very same door sharing stall space with you.

Excusing Health

"There is no excuse for that." How many times have you heard that in your lifetime? How many times have you said that very same statement? I admit that I have said that statement countless times and have been the recipient of it as well. I guarantee there is health in humility!

Anyway, while spending the evening running and then eating with my very close friend, I discovered the many ways we can find unexpected health in excuses.

Excuses get a bad rap. Making excuses seems synonymous with laziness, lack of responsibility, and an inability to admit when you are wrong. And to some degree, that is an accurate depiction of an excuse. But what often gets overlooked (and under-used in the English language) is that excuses allow us to experience wild adventures and enjoy abundant health... And giving us any reason to celebrate life is healthy.

My friend and I have an excuse to get together most Wednesday nights because we are training for a half marathon. Some might say that running is how we would experience our health, but to be honest, I often feel a little less than optimally healthy when I run! But the running is our designated time to catch up. So, as we huff and puff our way toward our weekly mileage goal, we experience the unexpected health that our excuse graces us with: friendship, connection, motivation.

Life seems to get busier and busier. We are all busy. Sometimes, we need to make excuses to give ourselves permission to take a timeout from the hamster wheel of our lives. I have an excuse for many essential necessities in my life: I make excuses to experience a place because there's just no excuse not to! I purposefully donated my coffee machine to my parents, so I have an excuse to have a quick morning cup o' Joe with my mom. And sometimes, I love to blame the weather for staying in and watching movies on a random Saturday (the weather is always an excellent excuse for relaxation).

We shouldn't need an excuse to have a little fun, catch up with friends, or unwind from our responsibilities, but if an excuse is the only thing that allows you to relax, then excuse away!

So the next time you make an excuse, make it a healthy one. And from this day forward, consider the positive, healthy usage of that word. Change your excuses to be less of a way out and more of a way in.

Selling Health

We are a nation of collectors, of hoarding, mass consumption, and buying. I wonder if any other country has as many Anonymous workshops as we do? I've seen advertisements for Hoarders Anonymous, Clutterers Anonymous, and Shoppers Anonymous... All useful classes to help people become aware of their insatiable appetite for collecting stuff.

Well, as my journey toward unexpected health continues, I have found, tucked in the back of my closets (next to the suits that I will never wear again), some important health insights in garage sales.

While digging through my collection of clothes, knick-knacks, and sports gear, preparing for this weekend's garage sale, I became acutely aware of the bargain price of unexpected health in getting rid of unneeded paraphernalia in our lives: it's free! And being able to experience vitality for no additional charge is healthy. In fact, garage sales will usually give you a little return on your health investment. Not only are you freeing your life of unwanted, no longer needed clutter that can cause disharmony and dis-ease in your life, but you may also be providing an item for someone in need. And let's not forget that gaining a few extra bucks in your pocket never hurt anyone, either.

Garage sales can be a lot of work. But for all the effort it takes to put one on, you can gain much more by the freedom you experience when your house (and your life) is eliminated from the clutter and chaos.

So the next time you feel your world is overcome with stuff, consider a garage sale a healthy and helpful option for peace of mind. It is one of the most lucrative health solutions you can give yourself.

Tripping Out on Health

Travel, both near and far, is passport-stamped full of unexpected health. Traveling allows us to visit old friends or make new ones (healthy? Yep!) and doing a bit of sightseeing opens our eyes to a bigger world (and we all know that is healthy). But the unexpected health in traveling is that when you get away from the consistency of your life, you are more aware of possibilities that come flying (or driving) your way, and finding opportunities in any zip code is healthy.

During my mini getaway to Boulder, I had more time to leisurely read, think, and explore. I was physically removed from my day-to-day surroundings, which allowed me to experience a new area. Just like my obsession with experiencing farmer's markets in various places, I also love immersing myself in a town's festivities, events, and culture. In many areas, local newspapers, magazines, even posters will elaborate on the happenings of the month… And Boulder was no exception. And what did I find right next to the weekend's event calendar? I discovered a magazine full of potential for creating my own passions.

Sometimes it takes getting away and a little R&R to see the opportunities back at home. It took me perusing the possibilities in a foreign town to realize the potential in my own.

So the next time you feel the need to get away, to travel, be aware of what you do, what you see, and what you read. You may be on a sightseeing trip, but you may return with a bag packed full of "souvenirs" for your growth... and your health!

A Health Bargain

One day I hosted a much-anticipated garage sale. At 7 a.m., we were out and ready to face the garage sale world, full of bargainers and thrifty shoppers. At 7:47 a.m. (the Craigslist ad said 8 a.m., but whatever), we had our first customer. And by 10 a.m., we had wheeled and dealt our way toward fortune... Okay, maybe more like ten bucks, but in that short amount of time, I discovered some unexpected health in bargains.

Earlier, I talked about the unexpected health in garage sales. But on that day, when selling our treasures for bargain prices, I realized that although we might sell our goodies to make a buck or two, what we can offer another is invaluable... And sharing the wealth of health is healthy. That day, I watched one of my close friends sell his dining room table, a sentimental piece for himself that he bargained down to sell at a below-market value price. At first, he seemed annoyed that he had allowed someone to buy such a memorable piece at such a bargain price. To top it off, my friend had to use his truck to deliver this piece of furniture to the couple's house... at no additional cost. After returning from the delivery, I witnessed a person who recognized someone in need and responded accordingly, whether knowing this person personally or not.

See, when we bargain with someone else, we have no idea what their story may be. We have no idea of their financial or familial situation or whether they may desperately need that piece of furniture, those items of clothing, those towels, sheets, or shoes. My friend's bargain gave these people an item to help start over, to re-create a home that they had just lost.

So the next time you make a bargain or are being bargained with, remember that everyone has a story. Your overly generous bargain may be giving another in need the gift of a new story... and of renewed health.

A Health Shoot

I wish I had a better eye for capturing beauty. I look at National Geographic and wonder how someone can be blessed with such an ability to create breathtaking experiences by capturing and developing a moment. Photography has brought me to tears. A captured moment has inspired change, and a simple black and white photo has spoken volumes to my soul. Today, while taking in beauty through my camera lens, I discovered the unexpected health of taking pictures.

I find it fascinating what we see through the lens of a camera. As I prepared for my salon's photoshoot one day, I took extensive time figuring out the best light, the most complementary angles, and the most profound scenery. I asked myself, "What do I want others to see in this space? What experience do I want others to have here?" Taking photos forces us to look for the most beautiful elements. It literally forces us to be aware of the beauty surrounding us... And being forced to see the magic that envelops us is healthy.

Even if you are a simple photographer like myself, the very act of taking a photo of a group of friends can inspire health. For me, taking a picture usually ignites a glance-around to see if there is a flower-filled backdrop, a sunset, or a beautiful work of art to stand next to or in front of. Isn't that part of turning an everyday picture into a captured piece of beauty, of health?

We are constantly reminded of the ugliness in our world, the pollution, the concrete parking structures, the garbage. But when we go behind the lens of a camera, our eyes are on the lookout for something beautiful, something inspiring... Something healthy! On that day, I saw the salon like I have never seen it. I have walked through the space countless times, but on that day, with a camera around my neck, my sight expanded. On any given day, I walked in looking for what needs to be improved, what needs painting, fixing, updating. But on that sunny Sunday, I came in looking for the light, for the best way to accent the archways, the paintings, the little details that made the salon unique and eclectic. And because I was looking for it, I found it.

So the next time you reach for your camera or are asked to take a picture for someone else, consider yourself a lucky candidate for capturing the beauty that surrounds you. Because as you catch a moment and create a still image, you are giving yourself the gift of health... And possibly capturing it for someone else!

A Healthy High

I used to be a questionably unhealthy adrenaline seeker. I loved fast roller coasters and crazy carnival rides. I even spent my tickets through the completely corny haunted house at the local fair. To my mother's disapproval, I have bungee jumped—three times—off of a questionable piece of machinery in Mexico. I have had my eyebrow pierced, my nose pierced (twice), and have the cutest little butterfly tattooed on my ankle. Although the tattoo actually has sentimental value, the rest of my thrill-seeking adventures have been met with familial disapproval. But one night, I received a big dose of adrenaline, the greatest upper, and of course, the unexpected health from getting high—on life, that is!

You know that feeling you experience from adrenaline? You have more energy than you know what to do with, you feel elated. Let's be honest, you feel *high* from whatever gave you the adrenaline rush. Oftentimes though, adrenaline highs come from potentially harmful influences, dangerous engagements, unsafe circumstances, drugs. But life and the people we are surrounded with can also give us the quick hit of adrenaline, a healthy life high. And discovering healthy ways of finding elation is healthy.

Life can be somewhat depressing at times, which is why it is so easy to be thrill-seekers, adrenaline junkies, and living-on-the-edgers. But sometimes, I wonder if we live in that sort of heart-attack-waiting-to-happen drama because we are missing some needed depth in our lives. I look back to when I felt the need to bungee jump and I can be humbly honest and say that I felt anything but fulfilled at that time. So I sought fulfillment in adrenaline. But now, I am learning that life and the people I am surrounded with feed my soul with a healthy high. My high did not come from a dangerous act of stupidity but from engagements with old friends, new friends, and soul friends.

Yes, life can be a downer. But life can also bring sustainable fulfillment when we douse our worlds with meaningful experiences, inspiring people, and health-promoting possibilities.

So the next time you feel the urge for a little adrenaline rush, consider the danger, the possible detriment, and the potential letdown you may experience after. Search out the longer, more sustainable highs that come from life and people. Be a life seeker, a change creator, and a health promoter.

Bottled Health

Our bodies are made up of over seventy percent water. Isn't that incredible? It's hard to imagine our insides floating around in such massive amounts of H2O, but it's true. Because of this fun fact (I'm not really sure how fun it is, but at least you'll have another answer the next time you play Trivial Pursuit!), it is clear that there are apparent, expected health benefits to water consumption. In a nutshell, water keeps your body lubricated. A little swig off your Klean Kanteen (quick plug for my favorite water container) can have your muscles, tissues, and ligaments functioning at optimal levels. Water keeps skin hydrated, which also keeps the wrinkles away, and of course, aqua helps flush toxins out of our bodies. But the less-than-obvious, unexpected, health benefit to water is that when you feel the need to hydrate yourself, rest assured you are participating in life... And being alive in this lifetime is healthy.

I went for a way-overdue run one day. During my run (with my four-legged friend, of course), I became acutely aware of two things: 1) I should run more, and 2) I was in dire need of some water. I had left the house without my water bottle, and forty-five minutes into the run, I was ready to lap up the rainwater on the side of the road. I made my way to my pup's favorite swimming hole so at least she could cool off and hydrate (with some questionable water, but oh well), but there was no rejuvenation for me, so away we went to complete our full-circle loop back home. Tap water never tasted so good!

But as thirsty and dehydrated as I was (which by the way, is *not* healthy!), I was also acutely aware of how alive I felt. When we are active in life, physically, mentally, spiritually, we actually become thirstier and water is a brilliant indicator of how alive we may be feeling. When I am engaged with life on multiple levels, I am thirsty for more. I want more connection, more meaning, even more water. And as we grow into ourselves, we better understand what our bodies need... And water happens to be one of *the* most vital nutrients we can ingest.

So the next time you are looking for a thirst quencher, consider water the most healthy choice you can give yourself. You are filling your body and your soul with a little liquid health.

Toys "R" Health

Advertisers are intelligent. The strategic placement of their products is usually brilliant. How easy is it to walk out of Target with *way* more than you needed simply because of the last-minute goodies in the one-dollar section? Or how many times have you bought gum from the basket on the Starbucks counter because you *know* you will have coffee breath after your beverage? And my personal weakness: Burt's Bees chapstick packs at the very end of the checkout line. I am usually pretty good at avoiding the last-minute purchases at stores—you know, the mini-me versions of sanitizing gel, travel-size lotion, and sugar-free gum. But one day, while in line and surrounded by every bouncy ball, paddleball, and endless candy assortments from Big League Chew to Now and Later, I discovered the unexpected health in toys.

Now before I go on, let me preface this post by saying that I am in no way advocating cluttering your house, car, and backyard with a bunch of plastic toys for your kids. I actually think the children of this generation have *way* too many toys than they know what to do with. I am pretty sure I was quite content with a few bowls and some mud or sand to play with. In fact, I am not even referring to children and toys today. I am speaking to the young-at-heart, those who love to play, and those who wished they played more.

Let's go back to my time waiting in line: as I stood staring at all of the junk moms have to creatively distract their kids from (advertisers can be cruel to parents sometimes!), I focused in on one toy—a harmonica. I snatched it up and made the healthiest two-dollar-fifty purchase I have made in a long time.

As soon as I got into my car, I cranked up my country music, took the harmonica out of its holder (yep, it came with a carrying case!) and began playing along with the music. Well, I wouldn't quite call it music, but it was noise! At that very moment, three things happened. First, an immediate Cheshire-cat grin adorned my face. Second, I was force to take deep, diaphragmatic breaths in order to blow out a turn. And third, I burst out into laughter.

If a toy of any age category can have these effects on you, then it must be healthy!

To be honest, I didn't care that I looked like a total crazy lady driving down the street with a green harmonica hanging off her lips, laughing to herself. I felt that child-like playfulness enjoying my little instrument—my toy. As I drove along, blowing out whatever melody I thought resembled the Tim McGraw song playing through my speakers, I thought about how great of a stress reliever this toy could be. If there had been traffic, I would never have noticed. I would have been merrily distracted by my harmonica playing. I wondered why harmonicas weren't being sold at car wash stations, drive-thru Starbucks, and Targets across the state. If only people knew what a stress reliever it could be.

So the next time you are shopping, think about the unexpected ways that a toy may help relieve stress and bring about health in your life. Maybe I just found the key to eliminating road rage, with one two-dollar-fifty harmonica at a time.

Healthy CliffsNotes

I have been wanting to do this unexpected health insight for a while. One day, as I stared at my computer screen, trying to condense my entire professional background into thirty to fifty words for my Livestrong bio, I finally found the reason to write about the unexpected health we find... when we get to the point!

Relaying information in the short-and-sweet, quick-and-dirty style is rather profound. Minimum word counts tend to drive a point home because people's attention spans can handle the five-minute, short-form tidbit of knowledge... And making a poignant impact in people's lives is healthy.

Information and impact can be lost when we are long-winded. People get bored listening to long stories. Even if the story is amazingly inspiring, the longer we blab about it, the less inspiring it becomes.

So the next time you feel the need to relay some useful information, some healthy knowledge, get to the point. Meaning does not require a lot of words. So use your words wisely.

Punching in the Timeclock for Health

I have had a decent amount of jobs in my life. Let's see, I have worked at a coffee shop, a teeny-bopper clothing store, I've worked for a rafting company, a bar, I've catered, I've worked at a fitness club (a few different times!), I have done inside sales, outside sales, I've been a director, an intern, and an owner. As I think back to the times when I wondered what in the world I would possibly do with my life, I discovered that there are endless amounts of unexpected health to be had in dead-end jobs.

It's easy to feel bad when you flip from one job to the next. Sometimes, it takes many years and many jobs to find our niche. But the unexpected health that punches in the timeclock while dabbling in multiple careers is that every job, every skill set, and every duty learned is a building block for our true calling in life. And being groomed to fulfill our utmost potential is healthy.

Once, while talking about a potential business opportunity, I found myself seeing how nearly *all* of my past jobs could help propel this business possibility into greatness. All of the times I questioned what I was doing, all of the moments I felt bad that I was not doing what I thought I should be doing (which is unhealthy!), and all of the jobs I worked and left, have all been crucial to my development. They have all been instrumental in creating the person I am today and the career I now have and love!

So the next time you feel stuck in a dead-end job, remember that where you are right now, today, is exactly where you need to be. Every experience we have is an opportunity to build on another. The job you may be dreading today is preparing you for your dream job in the future.

Birthday Betterment

Have you ever noticed that birthday cards become somewhat depressing as you age? As you get older, the jokes about memory lapses, sagging skin, and hair loss become boring and old. But as I prepared to celebrate the day one of my closest friends was born, I discovered the unexpected health in birthdays.

Now that my friends and I are no longer teens, it would be easy to dread our birthdays. As our age increases, so does our awareness about how fast life goes and how quickly our time here on this earth really is. But the unexpected health in birthdays and getting older is that as we grow older (I prefer to say "grow in"), our lives continue to be filled with lifers. Lifers are those special people that turn into non-blood-related family members. When we are younger, we tend to have more seasonal friends, high school friends, college friends, traveling friends, fun friends, sports friends. But the beauty, the health, of having a birthday year after year, is that you start to filter out those friends who are not necessarily meant to be by your bedside the day you die. Getting older gives us the permission to choose who we spend our time with, who we share our world with, and who we invite to our annual birthday parties.

So the next time you celebrate a birthday, if you are feeling sad about your age, forget about it. Remember that age brings about a certain peace of mind, and that those celebrating with you are probably some of your lifers!

Eat Out, Health In

Sunny Sunday mornings are priceless. To wake up and have the sunlight shining through your windows and then to go outside and feel the warmth on your face, elicits an incredible sense of health for *this* spoiled Californian. One of my favorite pastimes on a day like that is to take a stroll downtown. I love seeing all of the people out and about enjoying the weather and the fresh air. But one day, as I took a stroll with some of my favorite people, I discovered the unexpected health in going out for breakfast.

Now we all know about the importance (the health) of eating breakfast. This is the most important meal of our day. What we consume sets the tone for our energy level, our brain functioning, and our overall sense of health and well-being. But the unexpected health benefit of a good cup o' joe and an egg scramble while sitting outside is not only a healthy way to start your day, it is also a perfect opportunity to enjoy a little mentally stimulating community time. Plus having a place to go that offers physical and mental health is healthy.

On that day, as my friends and I squished our seven adult bodies into a table meant for four, we reminisced about our previous day's activities, talked about that day's necessities, and dreamed about the future's possibilities. What a great way to start anyone's day! How healthy it feels to nourish our bodies with healthy proteins, fats, carbs, and coffee while nourishing our minds, our hearts, and our worlds with good friends, sunshine, and potential.

Although any meal out can have these similar health benefits, weekend breakfast time is unexpectedly healthy because it tends to be the time of day when most of us function best to think clearer, dream bigger, and become greater.

So the next time you have the opportunity to go out for a weekend breakfast, don't pass it up. You just never know what a circle of friends, packed into an undersized booth or painfully small outdoor patio furniture, can create for each other. While you fill your bellies with food, you can be filling your hearts with joy.

Health in a Bottle?

I may ruffle a few feathers with this unexpected health insight. I am prepared to come against some resistance with my correlation between health and something that has caused much grief and sadness in lives, but bear with me, for my insight is not so cut-and-dry as it normally is. Because as I stopped and thought for a moment about conversations I have had both recently and in the past, I discovered the unexpected health in drinking.

Before you close this book, swearing that I have lost my mind (and my vision of health), let me explain. Social drinking can have *some* health benefits: a glass of red wine is actually heart healthy (nitrate-free please!). Going out for a drink with friends promotes community gathering and a cold beer and hot dog (I prefer bratwurst) at a baseball game once in a while isn't going to hurt anyone. But the unexpected health benefits of drinking is that alcohol can reveal the truth… And knowing the truth is healthy.

Let me delve in a little further. People drink for a variety of reasons, some healthier than others. Because alcohol is a depressant, it can heighten the emotional state of someone who is already feeling a little down. It can make someone who is already a little annoyed become really angry. Alcohol amplifies everything. What I noticed more recently is how alcohol is a permission slip of sorts. When we drink, it is almost as if we are allowed to feel the depth of whatever we are feeling... And oftentimes, we speak it too! And more often than not, when we speak our unfiltered feelings after a glass of wine (or two), we tend to get a straightforward, yet surprisingly comforting (and healthy) response.

To be honest, the unexpected health I am referring to more so than alcohol is that when we spill our guts, our innermost feelings, to those we love, we are oftentimes not disappointed. So why do we feel we need liquid courage to do so? Why does it take a few cocktails to reveal the depth of our emotions, our sadness, our fear, our frustrations? Are we worried about the response we think we'll get? Are we scared to speak the truth?

I propose we take our liquid courage and turn it into solid courage. Let's take all of the times we have laid our heart on the line and been vulnerable and relate to each other, minus the booze. Alcohol abuse is a big problem in our country. We rely on it too heavily as our excuse to act out, to reach out, to let off some steam, to get angry, and to get sad.

So the next time you feel a little extra sensitive or a little more emotional, try telling a friend, a loved one, the liquid courage version—minus the liquid. We cannot progress as a human race if we rely on external substances to move our mouths. Instead, we will find much more sustainable health, much greater communal depth, when we, as John Mayer tells us, "say what we need to say."

Doubting Health

I should buy stock in Merriam-Webster's Dictionary. I love looking up the meaning of commonly used words because sometimes, I want to make sure I'm spelling them correctly. Other times, I like to make sure I am using the word correctly in a sentence. But most times, I want to delve into the meaning of words, to pull them apart, dissect them a bit, and then, of course, try and discover the health that can be extracted from a word that may very well seem quite unhealthy.

Today's word of the day is: doubt. After researching this particular form of a verb and having an always humbling experience with doubt, I discovered the unexpected health in, no mystery here, doubt. When we doubt, we are assuming that the likelihood of something happening is nil. Essentially, we lack faith in other people, fate, and a greater purpose for our lives. I don't think I need to point out the unhealthiness of this form of "stinking thinking," as my mom likes to say. But the unexpected health that should ease our fears is that doubt is pointless to worry about, and eliminating unnecessary worry in our lives is healthy.

Doubt could be synonymous with stress, and stress is correlated with ill health. More often than not, our doubt is a futile use of the brain cells and stress hormones we use up when we think something will not work out. When I find myself doubting, I immediately feel a heightened sense of anxiousness and anger. I begin thinking about the conversation I'm going to have, the points I'm going to make, and the actions I should take to remedy the so-called problem. Well, as you can imagine, there is no conversation, no point to be made, and actually, no problem. Most times, my doubt is completely unjustified and uncalled for.

We waste a lot of our time and energy on situations that never happen, conversations we never have, and anger we don't need, all because we doubt. But as we become more aware of the pointless act of doubting, we can empty our minds of garbage (doubt, fear, distrust) and allow ourselves to be filled with potential. Having doubt limits our possibilities for our unique creative expression in this world.

So the next time you doubt a person, a situation or circumstance, leave the doubt at the door. Focus less on what *may* or *may not* happen, and instead, keep facing forward, knowing that as you keep walking this life with your faith shoes on, you have, "nothing to fear but fear itself."

Fact Checking for Health

You may have known this unexpected health tidbit was coming. I have mentioned the healthy aspects of this action in previous posts but today is the day to explain the benefits, the unexpected health, one finds in research.

When I was in high school, I distinctly remember doing anything to avoid research. I found any roundabout way to explain my point without going to the library (yes, the library—pre-internet dependence) and without putting the time and effort into exploration. But as I have grown in, I welcome the opportunity for a little investigative search for truth.

Now of course, there are many obvious health aspects to research: learning more is an empowering experience; you know, "Knowledge is power." Doing a bit of research allows us to better understand unknown places, cultures, and lifestyles, and of course, being a whiz at finding answers puts you on the fast track to expansion. But the unexpected health in research is that the more you discover, unravel, and comprehend, the deeper you are traveling into life... And living life at the point of depth is healthy.

Learning, just like life, can be taken at face value. You can go through life being mediocre. You can learn the CliffsNotes version of just about anything. But diving in and living and learning from a place of research, of inquisition, allows for profound growth and optimal health. As you dig in to find answers to the more meaningful questions and find more meaningful answers to life's simpler questions, you experience a heightened awareness within your surroundings.

So the next time you have the opportunity to discover a little more, to research, take your learning (and ultimately, your health) to another level...dig in and go deeper.

Unplanned Healthcare

I am what you call a planner. I am obsessively organized, highly cognizant of time, and extremely aware of schedules. My favorite iPhone app is, you might have guessed it, the calendar. My life revolves around the *dings* of my iPhone calendar reminders. But one night, as I had an unplanned, unscheduled, and un*ding*ed dinner date with one of my favorite people, I, actually we, discovered the unexpected health that pours onto us with unpredictability.

Let me set the scene: first of all, I was scheduled to do a six-mile run that day. My very planned but not always followed training calendar indicated what my evening *should* have looked like. But then, an unexpected surprise came: a dinner invitation. So I bagged the run and opted for a walk downtown with one of my best friends for some delectable Mexican food. As we walked, we felt the sunshine on our faces. We sat at a great little table and gabbed away... So healthy for so many reasons. We got the check, paid the bill, and headed for the door, ready to start our trek back to the house. But as soon as we opened the door, we noticed that our sunny weather had turned to a monsoon evening (in fact it was pouring!). Not only was it raining like cats and dogs' (I always wonder about this saying... What would it feel like to rain like cats and dogs?), the rain was enhanced by a forceful wind that made the raindrops slap your face and sting your eyeballs as you walked. There we were: me with a thin, cotton shirt and no jacket and my friend with a hoodless jacket and obviously, there was no umbrella around.

Enter unexpected health. As we stood under the awning, wondering who we could call to pick us up and drive us home while laughing at the craziness of this California night, I realized how unpredictably humorous life can be... And finding the lightness in life is healthy.

Life can be very heavy sometimes. Our lives can be rained on with stressors, hardships, sadness, and loss. These are sad experiences to deal with, live with, and function with. Sometimes I think God (or whatever Higher Being you believe in) uses humor, randomness, and unpredictability to keep us sane. Our unpredictable weather caused a chain reaction of laughter among those who didn't prepare, didn't schedule, didn't plan for the evening's forecast. And because of that, we experienced health... with laughter!

So the next time you have the opportunity to be spontaneous, last minute, and unprepared, do it! Life is too short to be so regimented, so live on the edge a little... Because in the edges, we find our growth and our health.

Unplugging the Earplugs Toward Health

This post is dedicated to all the light sleepers out there. That's right, the ones who travel with ear plugs, who require absolute stillness in the night, and who absolutely cannot share a room with a less-than-quiet snoozer. While you may lay awake at night, cursing the noisy loved one snuggling next to you, I have an unexpected health insight to share with you. This remedy requires no NyQuil, no Tylenol PM, and no other sleep aids. The only prescription this aid needs is a change of perspective, discovering that there is unexpected health in snoring.

Now, let me first say that I am actually referring to those listeners of the snoring, not the snorer themselves. I have quite a few friends who complain of having disrupted sleep because of their significant other's overwhelming intake of air throughout the night. Although one's sleep patterns may be temporarily compromised, having a snorer in your life is actually a healthy reminder that you are not alone... And knowing (and hearing!) that you are not alone is healthy.

As I laid in bed tonight, typing away in the silence of the night, I heard a small, muffled snore coming from the side of my bed. I looked to my right and curled up in her oversized, fit-for-a-queen bed was my dog, Lucca. Her little carob-chip-eyebrowed face was smooshed into the side of her bed and out of her caramel outlined mouth that makes her look like she's smiling, was a faint snore. I couldn't help but smile… Here was this little sacked-out dog, snoring the night away. What a life!

Snorers can be annoying, especially if you are a light sleeper. But when you hear a snore, it means you have a "someone". They may have two legs, they may have four, but what matters is that in the quietness of nighttime, when people oftentimes feel alone, even when surrounded by others, a healthy snore can jolt your memory, reminding you that you are not alone after all. That deep, sometimes obnoxious, intake of air can be the healthiest song to your ear because at that moment, you know you are surrounded by another.

So the next time you feel the overwhelming need to reach for your earplugs, just remember that the snorer next to you… is next to you. You are not alone.

Health Security

By now, you know very well about my struggles with waiting and have talked *ad nauseam* about the need to slow down, even stop, and pay attention to the beauty going on around us. But as I stood waiting, I discovered the unexpected health in security lines.

Ever since September 11, 2001, our airports, travel, even packing requirements have become a haven for all sorts of unhealthy behavior: people seem tenser, more on edge, and definitely more impatient the day they are traveling. You see people rolling their eyes at the person digging through their luggage, trying to find their passport. You'll notice the stink eye you get if you sound off the alarm when walking through security. You can just feel people saying to themselves, "How hard is it to remember to empty out your pockets before walking through!?" But the unexpected health that resides right alongside your personal belongings on the conveyor belt of a security line is that standing in that line means you are going somewhere... And being able to travel outside of your comfort zone is healthy.

Security lines and traveling can be frustrating. But for every minute waiting in line, every security checkpoint, bag check, and ID requirement, you are one step, one minute, closer to being on a plane, traveling to a destination other than your home address. If you are standing in the security line awaiting your vacation to start, then you have the health benefit of journeying toward relaxation, rejuvenation, and exploration. If you are going away on business, then you are blessedly healthy because you have a job. You may hate your job or hate that you have to travel for your job, but in an economy that experiences constant unemployment hikes and spikes, you are lucky.

So the next time you take a flight, remember that it is easy to see the glass half empty, to stress out over check-in lines, security lines, and bathroom lines. But when we step back and gain some perspective, I think we may take it easy on the person rifling through their belongings, emptying their spare change from their pockets, and removing their laptops in front of us. When we leave our own zip code, who knows what kind of possibilities we may encounter.

Tired of Health

As I sat thinking about the incredibly fun-filled weekend I had just had with one of my best friends, I could barely keep my eyes open. All I wanted to do is turn off the lights, roll over, and get some zzz's, in the hopes of recouping some of the lack of sleep from my weekend in Los Angeles. But as I lay here, typing away, eyes nearly shut, I discovered the unexpected health in being tired.

We often associate being tired with a slew of negative attributes: being tired can make people grumpy. When you're tired, it's easy to see the glass as half empty. And feeling the need for a little extra sleep can make it very difficult to find any health-filled motivation. But the unexpected health in being tired is that when you are tired, that means you have been active in life... And being an active participant in this lifetime is healthy.

Now of course, I am in no way condoning the hamster-wheel lifestyle where tiredness is overlooked and rest and rejuvenation take a back seat to forging ahead. But sometimes, we are tired because we were just having too much fun to stop and re-charge. That was the case that weekend: you take two girls who haven't seen each other in a very long time, add tons of sunshine, a convertible (to *really* let the light in), and fun places to go and interesting people to see, and what you get is a weekend where rest falls by the wayside... And that is perfectly okay!

Even though I was extremely tired that evening, I wouldn't exchange that for the world if it means I had a fun weekend with good friends. Life is short. Sometimes the most health*ful* experience we have does not come in the doctor-prescribed remedy. Yes, you should get your seven to eight hours of sleep every night. But you should also get your healthy doses of friend time, girls weekends, and living-for-today experiences.

So the next time you are feeling tired, think about the reasons why you are so beat. You may be physically tired and in need of some extra sleep... But in your lack of sleep, you may have gained some health.

It's all Greek to Me

Being the word geek that I am, I am always fascinated by the origin of these amazing little compilation of letters we call words. As I've mentioned in the past, I enjoy a quick peruse through Webster's Dictionary, unraveling the many uses of various verbs, nouns, and adjectives. But today, as I learned the deeper meaning of a word I often use, I discovered the unexpected health in words.

Words can and have caused unhealthiness at times. A damaging word can cause great pain in others. Words have been misused, creating slander, lies. Lawsuits and words exchanged in hate can cause division among families, friends, and party lines.

But the unexpected health in words is that as we uncover the origin of words (say, their Greek meaning), we can accurately describe ourselves, our world, and our feelings. And being able to articulate our human experience is healthy.

Let me explain. I have used the word "enthusiasm" (and "enthusiastic") time and time again. I love that word! I love it because it makes me feel happy and alive. But to be honest, I couldn't tell you the dictionary definition of it. So of course, I looked it up. Enthusiasm (noun): "absorbing or controlling possession of the mind by any interest or pursuit; lively interest." That sounds accurate, right?! But today, I was made aware of the Greek translation of "enthusiasm," which seems much more accurate. Enthusiasm: "The source of the word is the Greek *enthousiasmos*, which ultimately comes from the adjective *entheos*, 'having the god within,' formed from *en*, 'in, within,' and *theos*, 'god.'"

We often take words for granted. But for all of the years I have called people enthusiastic or have been called enthusiastic myself, I was really saying that I saw the god within them. That is so much more powerful, so much healthier, than being told that you have a "lively interest" in something.

I was challenged today. I was enlightened by words and the origins of which they were created.

So the next time you come across a word you use often but whose origin you're not completely sure about, I propose that you take some time and delve deeper into their meaning. Discover their origin, their many definitions, even their Greek translation. That way, the next time you refer to someone using a noun such as "enthusiasm," you will be able to share with them the honorable description you have blessed them with. Let us all use our words wisely.

Filling up the Tank on Health

Do you ever feel resentful when you have to bend over backward for people? You know, the people very accurately deemed "high maintenance?" I have had encounters with people like this time and time again, as we all have. I can get very annoyed having to jump through hoops and go out of my way for people who constantly need that extra attention. But one day, as I went out of my way to deliver a package to a delinquently paying tenant who doesn't even rent from us anymore, I discovered the unexpected health in taking the long way home.

The Dixie Chicks have a great song that talks about taking "The Long Way Around." They speak about the benefits of going about life the long way: approaching life differently than the average person, dreaming with your eyes open, living your life's potential—whatever that looks like.

I have always felt like I have taken the long way: I had numerous jobs while some of my friends found their career right away. I have dated a few fellas while others have been married for years. But on that day, I realized that it has been essential to take the long way around in my life, but it is helpful to take a long way home.

Let's get back to the package: I had been sitting there staring at this brownish-colored manila envelope for over a week now. I called the tenant to come pick it up, and day after day, it sat there. Finally, annoyed at having to go out of my way to call yet again, I picked up the phone, dialed, and after a quick conversation and to my surprise, was told that this tenant had cancer.

Sometimes I think we are pushed to go out of our way because we are guided to someplace, for someone. I was able to see this tenant today, tell her that I was praying for her healing, offering any words of encouragement that I could. I could tell she needed a friend, even though we have never really been friends. She needed a listening ear, a caring supporter, even a package deliverer. Yes, this delivery was out of my way, but I needed to be in her way, crossing her path on that day.

You never know how your day being inconvenienced might overwhelmingly enhance another.

So the next time you are asked or feel led to go out of your way for someone else, do it. Because although you may be required to take the long way home, your extra miles can create health for others, which in turn might be helpful for you as well.

In the Wee Hours of Health

I have referenced sleep throughout this health journey. I have talked about the health in wake-up calls and I have discussed the benefits of a healthy dose of sleep. But today, As I skipped out on my ideal sleeping hours (10 p.m. to 6 a.m.), I discovered the unexpected health of staying up late.

Now, I am not saying that being a night owl is the healthiest practice. In fact, there are quite a few unhealthy side effects to staying up into the wee hours of the night: I have talked about the health benefits of maintaining a fluid circadian rhythm, I have harped on the healthiness of getting seven to eight hours of restful sleep during specific hours (again, 10 p.m. to 6 a.m.), and especially for young ones, a healthy night's sleep during optimal hours is essential for brain development.

But staying up late every now and then can also have its place on the health charts because the unexpected health benefit to staying up late is that when time is limited, nurturing connection takes precedence over sleep… And valuing a shared experience at any hour of the day or night is healthy.

I stayed up *way* past my bedtime one night (it was actually the next morning that I finally went to sleep). But I stayed up late because my longest-term friend was in town for the night. Now of course, we could have said our hellos and hit the hay, knowing that we could catch up in the morning. But there was too much to talk about—too many stories, too many experiences, and too many exciting possibilities that needed to be shared... So we chatted away into the early morning.

Did I wake up tired? Yes. Did I arise and feel like I was operating at a little less than optimal functioning? Of course. But after a few hours' gab session, I felt rejuvenated in my soul. Although my physical body may not have had adequate rest, my heart and my soul were fully charged and ready to face the day.

Sometimes we need to make sacrifices in one area of our lives to fulfill more significant ones. I chose to lose a little sleep so I could gain a lot of connection.

So the next time you have the opportunity (and I do mean opportunity!) to stay up late and catch up with someone you love, do it. You can always sleep. You won't always have endless opportunities to connect.

Movie-ing Over for Health

Imagine: after a week of work, you come home on a Friday night, make dinner, and nestle in for a night of relaxation, of unexpected health, while watching movies.

There are lots of healthy aspects to watching movies. The main one is being able to relax and watch a good flick while turning off your mind. Another is watching a comedy to lift your spirits after a less-than-health-filled week. Watching movies is a perfect reason to enjoy a little crunchy popcorn... And chomping on these little puffs of deliciousness is a known tension-reliever.

However, the unexpected health that occurs when you press "Play" on your DVD player or catch up on your favorite Netflix series is that watching movies allows you to enter a world of fun-filled, inspirational stories. Stories inspire us and the storylines of both real-life individuals and well-written fictional characters are healthy.

Sometimes we need to check out: we need to think about something other than our own lives or just nothing at all. Movies give us permission to get lost in a character's life. But no matter how impractical or unrealistic movies can be, their stories can provide us with hope and expectations beyond our wildest imaginations. As I have said before, life can be heavy, stressful, and full of ups and downs.

So the next time you have one of those weeks, pop in a good chick flick, action film, or drama... It may be exactly what you need to feel a little inspiration and a little health.

Ordering a Side of Health

Friends play such a pivotal role in our lives. They help shape who we are, encourage us to become who we should be, and help us forget about who we are not. One day, after a long run with friends, I realized that there is unexpected health to be had in ordering take-out.

Now you might be wondering what take-out food and friends have in common. I began talking about friends and then decided to order up a round of confusion and talk about take-out food! Let me explain: ordering take-out gives us permission to take a short sabbatical from cooking (healthy? Yes!). Ordering from the to-go menu allows for a night at home minus the dishes (definitely healthy). And dinner in a box allows for more time to relax after a long day. But the unexpected health in take-out is that when you order in, you get unfiltered, unfluffed, and undazzled time with your friends... And having a night of PJs, playoff games, and pasta is always healthy!

Life doesn't have to be all or nothing. You can absolutely have your cake (in our case, Italian food!) and eat it too. My two close friends and I really wanted to hang out together that night. But, none of us felt like getting dressed up to go wait our turn for a dinner table, and then cram ourselves into a place to watch the Sharks game. So, we brought our desires home. We ordered take-out, turned on the game, and sat together, watching some hockey, eating some yummy food, and best of all, having lots of time for connection.

Take-out food provides a healthy opportunity to connect, especially if you don't want to go *out* to do it. As I've said before (and I wish I had come up with it myself), "You have to go in to go out." This is so true. We all need to be in the comforts of our own home, our own worlds, and our own skin in order to be out in this world. And sometimes, we need to be in, surrounded by our friends, to recharge and re-enter our environment.

So the next time you want to be surrounded and connected but have no desire to dazzle yourself for a night on the town, consider a night *in* with good friends and a great take-out menu, the greatest plate of health food you could buy.

Motherly Love

Mother's Day is a day set aside to appreciate those women in our lives who have taught us nearly everything we know: from manners to our ABCs and our 123s. But this insight is not about the significance of numbers. Although I am fascinated by the numeric system, on the day we celebrate all things Mom, I realized the unexpected health that is surprisingly found by being selfish.

Now, let me quickly clarify: I am in no way calling mothers selfish! Okay, I have that straight. Now back to the health.

Being selfish is not considered the most healthful attribute one can possess. There are healthy aspects of taking care of yourself, but to be labeled selfish is not something to be proud of. I should know, I have been called that before, and let's just say I *didn't* take it as a compliment! Moms are always giving and looking after their families. So Mother's Day is a reminder to see all the amazing work they have done and to take time to appreciate it.

My mom has always given of herself even when she appears to have nothing left. She always has leftovers in the fridge in case I have no food. She always has extra toothpaste if I need it, a spare set of sheets or towels, and a plethora of words of wisdom if I ever ask (and oftentimes, even if I don't ask!). No matter how old her children may be, a mom is always a mom... At least, that's what my experience has been.

I realize that I am incredibly fortunate. I know my mom's description may not match every other mom. But one of the most significant nuggets of knowledge (of health) that my mom has taught me is that selfishness has no place in humanity. Let me clarify: I am not talking about self-care practices such as speaking up for yourself, honoring your needs, and taking a time-out once in a while—which definitely has a place in humanity. I am talking about the think-only-of-yourself-and-your-needs mentality that creates disharmony and dis-ease in our world.

Our Earth is referred to as "Mother" for a reason. I believe the significance in this name relates to the self-lessness our Earth has shown us since the beginning. But we have not shown that same selfless behavior in return. I watched *Avatar* again one Mother's Day with my mom and family. I couldn't help but think about the giving nature of our Mother Earth—and my own mom! The health in self-ishness is only discovered when we realize how much more gratifying being selfless is! Being selfish on a day that cele-brates some of the most selfless people on this planet allows us to expand our lens, to be witness to what happens (how much healthier we feel) when we give as our mothers do.

So the next time you want a quick lesson in humanity, take a look at the mothers around you. It may not be your own mother, but remember, moms can be more than the women who birthed you. So look at the grandmothers, the godmothers, the stepmothers, the Earth Mother... They all play a part in raising selfless humans.

Signing Up for Health

The vast amount of unexpected health that stares us in the face is signs. Signs, those red, yellow, and green-colored metal objects that tell us, drivers, what to do, where to stop, when to go, and how to drive. What would we do without signs (besides getting fewer tickets)? We would live in a much more dangerous driving world without signs, that's for sure!

Signs are highly advantageous for our health on the highways. They are little protective indicators of what we need to do to remain the safest we can be on the roads. They provide common laws for all to abide by. Signs maintain vehicle flow with safe speed limits.

But the unexpected health found in signs is that these often bright-colored pieces of knowledge that stick out from the ground are constant reminders of how easy decisions can be when our eyes are open. And making our lives a little easier is healthy.

Let me explain: I am not saying that life is easy or that the decisions we make (or don't make) are no big deal. They're not. Life is not that black and white, or easy for that matter! But sometimes, what we should do or not do in life can be as easy as "Stop," "Slow Down," or even "Caution: Pedestrian Xing."

There are times in our life when we need to slow down, or stop for that matter. As I've said before, life can be crazy. Sometimes, a visual reminder to do what we need to do

So the next time you come across a sign on the side of the road, read it. And then, read between the lines. You just never know what avenue, what sign, or what form may be directing you. We can be guided by just about anything in life... And sometimes our signs are as obvious as just that.

Trimming the Hedges of Health

I was not born with the greenest of thumbs. Well, let me rephrase that: I may have a green thumb, but during my twenties and thirties, I never took the time to nurture a yard, a garden, even a small indoor potted plant! But as I grow in (or older, but growing in sounds much better!), I have found my love of creating beauty with a manicured landscape. And one day, as I trimmed my finally full-blooming climbing roses, I discovered the metaphorical unexpected health in pruning.

Now, for both plant and human species, pruning has many obvious health benefits: doing a little trimming allows for new growth to sprout, cutting the dead plant remains removes ugliness from an otherwise vision of beauty, and clipping away provides necessary nourishment for all things that thrive. But the unexpected health in pruning is that as you watch a plant flourish after being freed from unnecessary weight, you can find solace that you too will flourish from trimming away the unneeded in your life... And watching how cutting away creates health is healthy.

I watched as leaning, seemingly lifeless roses perked up as soon as I pruned away the "life suckers," those dead branches, dead rose buds, and leaves that suck the vitality out of any plant. But roses aren't the only species vulnerable to these "suckers of life"; humans are constantly surrounded and susceptible to such varieties. Have you ever let go of someone in your life and immediately (or shortly thereafter) felt lighter—literally? I have. My life path has encountered a few of these people, individuals who demand oxygen, energy, and vitality that suck me dry.

Just as we can visually see a rose bush flourish by pruning away what is no longer needed, we too will feel and see the health benefits of cutting free of those people who are "life suckers." If you wonder who these people are, simply pay attention to those who, when you leave their presence, leave you feeling depleted, exhausted, and sucked dry. Those are the suckers.

It is not to say that we will always feel wonderfully healthy and energetic in life, but if you pay attention long enough, you will recognize the ones who, more often than not, leave you feeling zapped of all vitality. These are the people who, if you used your clippers and did a bit of pruning, would allow your energy, your passion, and your zest for life return.

So the next time you are around someone and feel depleted, pay attention. Remember how you feel around them most times and act accordingly. Just because we love someone does not mean we are meant to have them in our lives forever. Sometimes, the healthiest act we can do is cut them loose.

A Healthy Character

I loved cartoons as a kid. I sang my heart out with Ariel in *Little Mermaid*, dressed up and pranced around the house like Alice in *Alice in Wonderland*, and desperately wished my dog would fit in my basket like Toto in *The Wizard of Oz*. Cartoons expanded my child-like imagination, allowed me to dream, even tested out my vocal chords (I have now resorted to singing only in the shower). But as adults, we are taught to leave the cartoons to the kids, to grow up and grow out of the free-thinking curiosity that make-believe elicits. But one day, at thirty-one years old, I discovered the unexpected health in cartoon characters.

Now, cartoon characters have instilled both healthy and not-so-healthy belief systems in people, small and tall. For example, princess characters have portrayed unhealthy body sizes and fairytale love stories that are both physiologically impossible and psychologically improbable to attain. However, these larger-than-life animated characters often display an exceptionally healthy outlook on an otherwise bad situation. But what I found most unexpectedly healthy about cartoon characters as I sat with the movie *Robots* playing in the background, is that real life can seem so unreal sometimes that we can only relate to it by watching the metaphors depicted through cartoon characters. And being able to relate through any storyline is healthy.

Let me explain: I find that cartoon characters often come across an internal battle. Think back to some cartoon characters: Ariel wanted to be human, Aladdin wanted to be great, Peter Pan refused to grow up...

All of these characters sought out adventures to discover their greatness. Sometimes, they actually found greatness by becoming something more than they were before they started on their journey. But most times, these characters realized that they already had this greatness inside of them... They merely needed the proper setting for the magic to unravel.

So the next time you watch a cartoon, remember that cartoon characters always tell that story about the life processes we all go through: questioning ourselves, traveling down various paths searching for our truth, and often finding out that where we are and who we are becoming is exactly what is supposed to be. But we need the journeys. We need to be a fish out of water sometimes. We need to take that magic carpet ride, and we need to take a trip or two down a rabbit hole. But what we find when the adventures are over, when we are back home in Kansas, is that our healthiest selves are who we already are, who we've always been. Maybe we just needed a little fairy godmother or a little pixie dust to remind us.

Cardstock of Health

I am a sucker for inspiration books. I have piles of flip-through pages of motivating sayings, mind-blowing stories, and amazing analogies. Unfortunately, there cannot be too many of these small, often square-shaped compilations for change in my house. And one day, after under-appreciating a franchise for years, I discovered the vast amount of unexpected health stuffed into the envelope in a Hallmark store.

Now, I don't know if there are still a lot of Hallmark stores around. So I am using Hallmark as a blanket name for card stores. I have often found myself leaving a card store with a tinge of irritation. "That'll be $15.78," says the cashier. What? For two birthday cards? It is easy for me to find the ill-feeling in the prices of a good old anniversary, sympathy, or birthday card. But what I have failed to give credit to is that card stores stock themselves with inspiration, and knowing the hot spots for a health recharge is healthy.

Think about it: what is one of the first places you think to go when looking for a meaningful gift? My guess is that Walmart does not pop into your mind (or maybe it does?!). However, Hallmark stores have it all. They have glass apples that say "#1 Teacher" for teacher appreciation week. They have statues of mothers and children for Mother's Day. And of course, they are stocked to the brim with inspirational books, plaques, and coffee mugs. These are all used as wonderfully healthy reminders of our and others' unique contributions to this world.

Our world needs more of these inspirational storefronts. Unfortunately, we have plenty of disease-promoting reminders. Take, for example, our beauty magazines, which often make people feel ugly (quoted from the pages of one of my favorite inspirational books, *Wear Sunscreen*). We need to shift focus away from all of the things we "aren't" to a focus of how wonderfully complete we all are. We need supportive environments that praise our unique gifts, our contributions, and our grace.

So the next time you feel the need for a little extra TLC, check out your local card store or mom-and-pop gift shop. You never know what sort of inspiration, motivation, and health may be awaiting your visit in the center aisle.

Pushing out the Parameters

I am surrounded by motivation in my life. As you now know, my decor consists of a lot of colors and even more inspiration. I have found (and I have read repeatedly) that to become what you are intended to become, daily reminders are vital to your expansion, hence the countless motivational sayings that grace my walls, fridge, and dishware. But after attending a transformational workshop, I discovered the unexpected health in mentors.

Now, I find it hard to say anything unhealthy about mentors. These thought-provoking, inspiring, and expansive individuals are encouragers for our lives. They help flush out our gifts, guiding us toward the most health-filled directions. And of course, mentors are people we can look to for strength when we feel too small to elicit significant change. But the unexpected health in mentors is that these people push us around, and surprisingly, being pushed around can be healthy.

First and foremost, please do not get confused with the health benefits of being pushed around. Of course, it is not healthy to be accosted by someone. But when we are flexible enough, moldable enough, we can be healthfully pushed toward health, and mentors are the perfect people for the pushing job. It is easy to get stuck in the story, you know, that old song-and-dance that we unconsciously tell ourselves, the story that keeps us stifled from experiencing greatness? We all have them. Some have stories about never being successful; others create stories about never living up to expectations; some have a paperback about their inability to ever be loved or get what they want. These are fictional accounts of limitations we create for ourselves. They are not true and they are not who we are. But we easily forget this and fall into the trap of believing the lie. Enter the mentors.

Mentors push you beyond your comfort zone. They challenge old belief systems, patterns, and ways of living. They see potential and inspire those around them to put on the sunglasses of truth to see the world and ourselves in an accurate light.

So the next time you are searching for some truth, some guidance, or even a good push in a healthy direction, get your mentor(s) on speed dial. They may push you around a little but know that the direction they push you toward is probably exactly where you need to be heading.

To Say No is to Know Health

I recently attended a sustainable business workshop. I sat, listened, shared, and participated in conversations about business practices I had never heard of before. I was enthralled by the tools I was given to empower myself as a business owner. I had attended workshops before and left with pages of notes, handouts, and pamphlets, only to go home, file them away, and never look at them again (unless I do some file cleaning). But as I put the preaching into practice, I discovered the unexpected health in saying no.

Saying no may come easy to some people. For you lucky souls, I commend you on your ability to speak up. But for many of us yes people, saying no has the same effect as nails on a chalkboard—ouch! Us yes people find it terribly difficult to say no because we are caretakers. And although there is nothing wrong with taking care of one another, when another's care takes constant precedence over our own, dis-ease and ill-health usually follow. This leads me to the unexpected health tidbit of the day: a no coming from the mouths of those who always say yes actually creates a yes situation... And empowering ourselves and others to find the yes situations in life is healthy.

Let me explain: when we actually say no, we are giving and receiving empowerment. We are creating the opportunity for ourselves and others to say yes to personal responsibility. I'll give you an easy example: a friend who works in a particular organization asked for my business to be a part of that organization... And I really didn't want to. Now for this yes girl, it would have been easy to say, "Oh sure," and then resent the hell out of myself for saying yes and resent the friend who asked me because I felt obligated to help her out. Well, I practiced one of my workshop tools and said no.

After the initial shock of my direct (but kind) refusal, I felt empowered. Of course, I had empowered myself by speaking my truth right away, without hesitation. But I choose to think that I also empowered my friend by stretching their comfort zone in sales. It's easy to ask a friend for a favor—or in this case, a sale. But how much healthier do we feel when we close the deal on someone we have no ties to? As salespeople, how much empowerment and pride do we have in ourselves and whatever we may be selling when we can engage a complete stranger in our product or services?

We need to be stretched in life. We need to step out of our comfort zones and, to borrow the phrase, "play a bigger game." The big game of life has many yeses and nos... And the easier time we have at letting go of what yes and no means (i.e. it's not personal), the greater empowerment we will have as a human race.

So the next time you feel the burning desire to say no, practice it. Be firm in your answers and know that as you say no a little more, or yes a little more (if you're a no kind of person), you are a part of empowering our world. Say yes to that kind of empowerment whenever possible... because in the nos, we will find the yeses.

Healthy Lip Service

Fashion changes with the weather. One minute you are wearing flared leg jeans, the next, skinny jeans. For a blink of an eye, wedge heels are the new must-haves and then before you know it, it's back to stilettos. Along with fashion, makeup takes a turn at keeping us confused consumers. Do I wear purple eyeliner or blue? Is matte finish *in* this season, or should my face look squeaky-clean shiny? Not that I follow the fashion or makeup trends (I'm lucky if I even wear eyeliner!), but I did discover some unexpected health today in lipstick.

Lipstick is another fashion *in* and *out*. Sometimes, the newest Glamour Magazine tells us we should be wearing the dark-lipped look of lipstick. Other times, lip gloss is the way to go. For the last few years, I have steered away from all lipsticks. In fact, I barely own any, and those I do own, I never wear. One of the reasons is that most lipsticks contain harmful, unhealthy ingredients that can cause a variety of health concerns (see *http://www.cosmeticsdatabase.com* for more on that topic). As I have grown in, I prefer to buy more sustainable products, limiting my lip color selection to a few fruit-infused glosses. But the unexpected health that one finds with lipstick is that this little twist-up lip art makes perfect proclaimers of your intentions… And having outlets for displaying your health is healthy.

I put my lipstick to work. I did not use it on my lips but instead made a declaration on my bathroom mirror, using the most perfect shade of reddish-pink (MAC calls it "Verve"). This name, of course, prompted me to look into the definition of "verve," which I found out means "enthusiasm, liveliness, vivaciousness."

Unused makeup, such as lipstick, can do more than sit in a drawer and dry out. My Verve, way-too-dark-for-my-face, lipstick became a pencil for me to express my liveliness about… life! I could have kept that old lipstick in my drawer, thinking that one day I might actually dress up for Halloween and need that exact lip color, but instead I wrote an affirmation for my eyes to see every morning, every evening… actually, every time I walk into the bathroom.

So the next time you clean out your makeup bag (or in my case, drawer), consider keeping your never-used lipstick. You just never know when you may need a unique, yet health-promoting writing utensil to encourage you on your health journey.

Letting Health Go

I can have a tight grip on life. Some have labeled that controlling, but I prefer to think of it in a more positive light, more like persuasive?! How about nudging? Okay, I may be a downright control freak, but rest assured that I am quite aware of my areas of weakness. And as always, I was humbly reminded of the unexpected health one finds when letting go.

Now, there are lots of apparent health aspects to letting go. Letting go allows faith and hope to make an entrance in any situation. Practicing the art of letting go makes way for unexpected opportunities to present themselves. Letting go frees up our minds, allowing us to focus on something more profound—healthier.

But the unexpected health in letting go is that as we loosen our grip on the outcome of our lives, as we blur our vision on what we think we know for sure, we actually gain more clarity... And having our vision cleared is healthy.

Recently, I wrote a "letting go" email, a just-need-to-get-this-off-my-chest kind of correspondence. As soon as I clicked "Send," I was pleasantly (and healthfully) surprised by the response I received. Then as I let go and sent my concerns out into cyberspace, I received the most uncontrollable but most gratifying gift—support.

I am constantly amazed at how letting go allows us to help gently loosen the tight-fisted grip we may have on the future of our lives. It is so easy to hold on for dear life, trying to force one outcome or another. But when we let go, we open the door for what is *supposed* to happen, not what we *think* should happen. I'm not saying that letting go answers all of life's mysterious questions, but I do find we can see a bigger picture. We can expand our lens just a little wider when we let go.

So the next time you find yourself trying to control a situation, throw your hands back from the death grip you are holding and allow for the magic to unfold. I am convinced that the more we let go, the more we let in.

Inspiring Health

Life is often profound. Circumstances, people, even seemingly random encounters all seem to correlate, integrating life's lessons and *aha*'s along the way. I have discovered that nothing is random in life. Every experience, every friendship, every relationship gone sour, all play a unique instrument in the orchestra of our experience on this planet. I discovered the unexpected health we feel when we are inspired!

If you haven't noticed by now, I am inspired by many things in life. My family constantly inspires me. My parents continue to amaze me with their giving spirit and undying role as cheerleaders. My brother will call on any given morning to warn me about the motorcycle police radaring cars, ensuring that his baby sis won't get a ticket. My friends cause a near jaw-dropping reaction by the inspiration I receive from their hearts and their work in this world. Nature inspires me, Hallmark cards move me to tears, even my dog causes inspiration now and again (actually, she is one of my greatest teachers).

As all of you know, being inspired has an abundance of health benefits: there is an endorphin-releasing quality when we are inspired, tapping into enthusiasm and energy we never knew we had. Having inspiration in our lives creates purpose when we question whether we have a reason for walking around on this planet and being inspired sets the bar for our life's work, igniting a spark of motivation to achieve our goals. But the unexpected health in being inspired is that when we feel that heart-tug pouring out of our beings, we can be led to do wildly unimaginable, oftentimes thought crazy, feats… And acting outside of the box is healthy.

Being inspired often eliminates the fear that keeps many of us from greatness. When we feel less than inspired in life, we can find ourselves in a place of stagnation, of looking around at our lives and feeling that yearn for something more, something rich, something profound. Inspiration jolts us out of that space. It's not that we are supposed to go through life constantly inspired, but inspiration and motivation jumpstart times that need a push in the health direction.

One day I was inspired. I was inspired as a good friend stepped up to the health plate of giving. I was inspired by the words of someone facilitating a paradigm shift in other parts of the country. And inspiration filled my heart when I looked at my plaque that reads, "What would you attempt to do if you knew you could not fail?" and my answer was a liberating, "Anything I dream of" proclamation.

We are often our own worst enemy. We can be our own worst critic, our biggest naysayer, and our toughest judge. But being inspired somehow silences that negative voice inside us. And if only that harsh voice is silenced for a moment, it is time enough to be witness to the power of possibility, to the potential we all have, and to inspiration.

So the next time you feel a little stagnant, a little stuck, look for inspiration. It is out there, ready to be discovered, embodied, and expressed in this world. Don't be scared when you feel inspired… Take a leap of faith and soar.

Wrong Wellness

I was never a know-it-all. Yes, I did pretty well in school, and yes, for the most part, I got along with my teachers. But I was never the kid who sat in the front row waving my hands in the air in the hopes the teacher would call on me. For any of my readers who were that kid, I am not making fun, just explaining my school day demeanor.

But as I have grown up (I use "up" instead of "in" very intentionally), I have become somewhat attached to being right. As I have disclosed in previous posts, I drag my soapbox along with me quite often, just in case I find a perfect little opportunity to spout out my thoughts, ideas, and beliefs—all of which, of course, I think are right! But one day, I managed to find a moment in which to profess my truths... And to my humbling yet profound realization, I discovered the unexpected health one finds in being wrong.

Being wrong can have all sorts of unhealthy qualities: being wrong directionally can cause one to get lost in life, being wrong about a person's character can cause great pain in another, and being wronged has its own laundry list of hurtful aspects. But the unexpected health in being wrong is that as we can admit when we are not all-knowing, we free ourselves and others from lies... And being set free from unhealthy belief bondage is healthy.

Just to reiterate, I said *lies*—you read that right! When we are obsessed with being right, making others wrong, we are spreading lies, and lots of them! The first lie is that there is always an absolute right and an absolute wrong. This is followed by the lie that we self-*right*eous people feel the need to always have all of the answers to the questions in life. We don't, can't and won't ever possibly be able to seek out and know even one millionth of the answers to life's questions.

The second lie relates to those always deemed wrong. Who says who's wrong? We righteous know-it-alls do! Being right or wrong, in most cases, is completely subjective and yet, we have made these objective polarities. Two people may have entirely different approaches to life... So who is right? Neither are. Both are. Because, what I continue to discover on my health journey is that what is acceptable and desirable for one person may be completely unacceptable and undesirable for another.

I recently got caught up in being right—and I was very wrong. My proclamation of rightness could have (and probably did) make another feel small... And that is a lie. I lied that day. No one is small. And just to be clear, I am in no position to make claims that I know what is best for anyone else besides myself. We have our own answers, we know our own truths.

So the next time you feel the need to prove your point and be correct, zip it! You don't know what is best for anyone else unless you walk in their shoes. You'll never know what it might be like to walk in a pair of shoes that are already spoken for. So let's allow freedom in each other. Freedom to try our own shoes on, to walk around, fall down, get back up. Life is hard enough just keeping our own lives on a healthy path... So admit your self-righteousness, and after that, admit that you were wrong. There's quiet freedom when we can let ourselves and each other off the hook.

Gusts of Health

Northern California can get pretty windy. Gusts of whirling air sometimes seem to blow through the trees outside my house, as if the branches were knocking on my window, commanding my attention with their tap, tap, tapping. As I was running over the Golden Gate bridge, surrounded by exquisite beauty and amazing friends, I was blown away by the unexpected health we can find in wind.

The music group Scorpions knew early on about the health benefits of wind: the feeling of excitement and anticipation that whirls through all of us when the wind blows, when it tousles our hair and our lives, the energy of the dreamers, the future innovators, and the wide-eyed explorers. And of course, as the song so magically reiterates, wind creates change. But the unexpected health that rattles our bones with the wind is that when we are blown around by the gusts, we are reminded about the fluidity of life... And physically experiencing the flow of life is healthy.

As anyone who has ever walked, run, or biked across the Golden Gate bridge knows, it is windy! The absence of wind barriers makes it a prime spot for experiencing wind. As I took in the beauty of the Bay and the city, I was taken aback (literally!) by the strong presence of the wind. It physically moved me. The gusts slowed me down, moved me from side to side, and blew my hair around.

The wind is a perfect metaphor for life. We experience all sorts of gusts in our lives: gusts of happiness, tornadoes of hardship, and windy times of the unknown. We can get blown around in many directions, but no matter which way we end up when the wind stops, it's a new perspective, it's a new landscape, and oftentimes, it's a wider lens.

So the next time the wind blows, step outside and experience it. Don't fight to stay in one place, just let it guide you. When we are open to the opportunities in life (the health) there's no telling where the wind will take us. But rest assured you will not stay stuck in the same place.

Roundtables of Health

The internet is a weaver. Somehow through its algorithms, the internet finds a way for us to be reacquainted with long-lost friends or help us find that exact thing we knew we needed but forgot what it was called. As I was checking my Gmail account, I discovered the unexpected health in networking.

Now, there are lots of obvious health aspects to networking: being in a network creates a sense of community, networking broadens our pool of friendships and colleagues, and of course, networking often generates potential jobs. But let me just say, I really don't enjoy networking. BNI and business mixers make me want to run in the other direction. But the unexpected health one finds in networking is that keeping in touch with people from all walks of life can pleasantly become part of maintaining the cyclical nature of our lives... And keeping our lives moving in a continuum is healthy.

A while back, I received an email from someone I worked with in the past. I hadn't thought of this person for a while but had always maintained a connection with them after I stopped working. So as soon as I saw her name in my email inbox, I had an immediate smile on my face because

I discovered another turn in the circle that is my life—a connection.

Networking creates hope. Hope creates action. Action creates expansion. Expansion facilitates health. The network that I had created with this person more than a year ago is now re-entering my life at a time I find to be quite non-coincidental.

You just never know what, when, how, or why people come into our lives. Sometimes they flutter in for a moment of time, eventually leaving, never to return. Other times, people blip into our space, and then make a reappearance again, at a different time and place in our lives. That is the beauty and the health of networking. The more we are open to possibilities, the more we take care of one another along our journey, the more we leave the door open for people to flow through our lives.

So the next time you make a connection with another, be sure (to borrow the phrase) "to leave them in good shape." Be gentle with people; be kind to those in your life. If you part ways, be sure to do so in love and with great care. You just never know when your paths may cross again, paving the way for a healthy reunion.

Pouring a Healthy Glass of Whine

I like to think of myself as a positive person. Now, of course, I have my days when I see the glass half empty instead of half full... There are even days when I can't even see a glass! There are times when the world seems full of opportunity, potential, and expansion, and other times when nothing seems to be going my way. But recently, as I found myself spouting off sentences of negativity, I discovered the unexpected health one finds when complaining.

It's hard to believe there is actually health to be had in complaining. But for all of you (myself included) who have ever complained in the past, fear not... You have the opportunity to experience abundant health with your complaints. As unhealthy as complaining can be—the negativity, the pessimism, the intolerance—when we complain, we are given a choice... And having the opportunity to choose health in life is healthy!

When we complain, we are pointing out something that is wrong, or awry, with *our* lives or circumstances. Our complaints may appear as if we are whining about a person, a job, or a situation, but really, all of our negative thoughts spewed out as a complaint are merely reflections of our own wants and desires. When we complain, we can use that as a verbal cue to pay attention to the deeper meaning present in our wallowing. What are we searching for? What is missing?

A complaint is really the wrong C-word... When we complain, we are actually comparing. We are saying that we are not satisfied with where we are, what choices we have made, or what may be lacking. But when we find ourselves complaining, we are immediately given authority over our own lives to remedy the complaint we are having. If we are frustrated with another, we can open our mouths and speak our truth. If we are unsatisfied with our jobs, we have the ability to facilitate a healthier experience or begin searching for a job better suited for us.

Everything in life is a choice. We choose what we talk about, think about, and act upon. Even when we complain, which is not the most helpful use of our time, we can experience health by taking action toward positivity, acceptance, and gratitude.

So the next time you find yourself complaining, take a moment and consider the shift of perspective available to you. We are all empowered individuals, able to experience health... Even in the midst of a good old-fashioned whine-fest.

Health on the Verizon

Technology has changed our whole world, from how we see it to how we communicate with it. I don't know one person who does not own a cell phone. I know people who don't answer their cell phones or always forget to charge them. I know people who are always on their cell phones, getting off a call, texting, emailing, playing games... You name it! We have become a cell-phone-crazy group of characters. Not only have we become cell-crazy, but phone manufacturers have also created a smorgasbord of activities for us to do on our devices, which has truly created a phone phenomenon. But as I used one of my iPhone's favorite features, I discovered the unexpected health in camera phones!

Now you might think that smartphones have much cooler apps than its standard camera. You might also say that camera phones have created a whole slew of problems, which they have. But the unexpected health in a camera phone is that your ability to have a camera on-hand 24/7 means you are able to capture the moments in life... And being able to share what visually touches our hearts is healthy.

Photos have this heart-tugging ability to move me, sometimes to tears, sometimes to laughter, sometimes to overwhelming grief. I can experience a whole gamut of emotions through one single still frame. The problem is, who schleps their cameras around with them anymore (unless of course they are a photographer)? Camera phones fill the need to leave the camera bag at home. They are the best little portable creation!

The moments in our lives happen at sometimes the most random of times, in the most unexpected places (just like health!). When these moments arise, we can capture them, allowing us to seize that moment, take it home with us, and reflect back when we need to. Whenever we want to return to that time, that moment, all we need to do is scroll through the pictures on our camera phones. And to really spread the health around, technology has given us this amazing gift of global sharing, allowing our moment to be another's as well.

So the next time you complain about your high phone rates, your expensive smartphone or the bulkiness of your new iPhone or Android, remember that in your pocket or purse, you hold a little piece of health just waiting to capture a little inspiration, a little moment. Use the gadgets on your cell phones, take lots of pictures, send them to your friends. Let's all create snapshots of health.

OCD:
Organizing Creates Delight

Anyone close to me knows about my preference for organization. Oh please, who am I kidding? I am borderline OCD when it comes to being organized. I just can't help myself. I love to leave a place with everything in order. That way, when I return, I feel an immediate sense of ease because I don't have to walk into a disaster zone. The more peaceful the environment, the more peaceful I feel.

Being organized has both health-promoting and health-depleting qualities. Organizing allows us to locate items we are searching for easily. But being obsessed with organization can cripple us from getting anything done because nothing gets done if it isn't done perfectly! On the other hand, having an organized spirit allows for a greater capacity to juggle multiple tasks at once. Still, oftentimes, that juggler becomes inundated with projects because "they're such a good organizer."

As you can see, being organized is a mixed bag. However, I think that there is one main unexpected health insight in being organized. As you make healthier use of your time by coming up with some sort of system to keep things organized, you are giving yourself a gift of possibility. And of course, being blessed with gifts in life is healthy.

When we are organized, we are freed up from the shackles that keep us from realizing our fullest potential. Being bogged down with playing catch-up, is like lacing up our running shoes and running a marathon. That feeling of exhaustion from physical exertion is much like the mental depletion we experience when catching up. Think about that term, "catching up." Even the words are exhausting. Having to catch up implies that we are chasing after something. What is that we are trying to run to? Why are we so far behind?

Being organized ends the game of self-defeat... At least as best as it can. I don't think it is realistic to expect that we will ever feel completely *done* in life, and that's a good thing. We should always want to be more—although preferably not more busy, more stressed, or more tired. Organization allows us to be more free, more open to possibility, and more able to take health-promoting journeys.

So the next time you feel a little less than organized or obsessively too organized (yes, that's possible!), start taking some baby steps toward a middle ground. Let's save the exercise for fun physical activity instead of dis-ease promoting defeat of trying to catch up. In the end, there is no race. So set the pace for your own sense of well-being. Start with a little organizing.

To the Nines... of Health!

I am a pretty casual girl. I love a good, comfy-fitting pair of jeans, cozy shirts, or tank tops, and I choose not to survive without my flip flops. That is the type of person I have become. Very rarely will you find me dressed to the nines and that is perfectly okay with me. But as my friends and I dressed up for an overrated movie, I discovered the unexpected health in dressing up.

Now of course, when we dress up, we can feel quite healthful: when we dress in professional attire, we often feel a little more confident in our adult bodies. We have an extra swagger in our walk when we are wearing a complimentary pair of heels, we feel a little more attractive when our outfit is an above-average ensemble of bright colors and original style, and dressing up makes us feel that certain specialness of an evening. But the unexpected health in dressing up is that when we bring out our physical best, we are also reminded of our emotional best... And letting our internal and external beauty shine is healthy.

Before I owned my hair salon, I rarely dressed up. I worked in an environment and went to school in a setting that had no dress code except for comfort. Because of that, I got very used to wearing the most comfortable outfits (and not always the most flattering ones). But since I have started working in the beauty industry, I have felt the desire to dress up a bit (and anyone in the beauty industry knows that you cannot run a business looking like a surfer chick). And on this particular girl's night, I had the opportunity to dress up again, to show off my creativity with my clothing.

When we dress up, we are taking pride in who we are. We are showing the world our creative gift of clothing compilation and color coordination. It's not that we should aspire to wear suits on a daily basis, but when we have the opportunity to spruce it up a bit, we should take it! Because as we spruce up our physicality, we take pride in what we present to the world. No matter what people say, our physical presence in the world *is* what we use as a canvas to display our internal world. Our outward care oftentimes reflects our internal care.

So the next time you have the opportunity to dress it up a bit, do it! Take the extra time to wear a little funkier outfit, bedazzle in a sparkly piece of jewelry, or show off those legs with a funky pair of wedge heels. Show the world who you are—inside and out!

Soul Searching for Health

I have talked more than once about my past serial monogamy. From the time I was very young, I have always had a boyfriend. I never allowed myself more than a few months to be single. After a breakup, I would work to claim my next victim—er, I mean boyfriend. All joking aside, I wasn't a *bad* girlfriend (some exes may disagree), I just lacked the ability to be okay without having my arms locked in with another. But as I sit on my deck, rocking back and forth on my patio furniture, typing away without a care in the world, I am reminded about the overwhelming healing, the unexpected health, one finds when single.

Being in love and being in a relationship has so many health aspects I wouldn't even know where to begin. In fact, I think that humans are meant to be in community and in relationships during our time here on this Earth. Being in a relationship allows our hearts to experience unexplainable joy. Having a special someone gives us a shoulder to cry on, a companion to share life with, and a last call at the end of any night. Many people are so scared to be alone that they will do just about anything to be attached to someone else. I have been one of those people. But during my several-year stint of singlehood, I saw where having time with no one but myself gave me clarity that continues to amaze me. And having a clear self-portrait is healthy.

For all of you singles out there (actually, even those in relationships may relate), let me share with you some of the more healthy insights I have learned based on sayings I have heard over the years:

1. Eggs thrive when dispersed in multiple baskets, so don't put all of yours in one.

2. Pedestals are never meant for another to reside on, so don't set your honey up there... They are bound to come tumbling off.

3. It does take two to tango, but it takes individual strength to learn how to dance.

4. The phrase "you complete me" is complete crap... We are never complete while we live in these bodies, in this place, and during these times. Our imperfection, our incompleteness, keeps us reaching for meaning, and that is good thing.

5. "For better or for worse" is more than just a saying we repeat after our pastors, priests, and ordained ministers. These words are not to be taken lightly. If your loved one's "worse" is a non-negotiable for you, then don't walk down that aisle... Walk away.

6. "I can't live without you" is actually a clear-cut sign that you should. Do not consider this a compliment when someone says this to you or you to them. It is a red flag that a relationship is based on need instead of love.

7. Love Potion No. 9 is poison. The myth that you can drink a magical tonic and fall in love with anyone is toxic. Don't force yourself to love and be with someone simply because you are afraid there is no one else... There is!

After the fear subsides, being alone gives us permission to inquire within, to do a little soul searching, a little self-investigation, and a lot of helpful self-care. I am not suggesting that these inquiries are impossible to do in a relationship, but oftentimes, we can become so deeply enraptured in the relationship that we forget that along with a "we," being in relationship still needs a "you" and a "me."

So the next time you find yourself at a time of single-hood, embrace it! Do not be afraid of being without a special someone. Consider your time as a single soul a perfect opportunity to learn more about another special someone—yourself!

Getting into the Health Business

Medical practitioners are not the only ones in the health business. You've got your farmer, your therapist, your natural foods store owner. Then there's the acupuncturist, the herbalist, and the health writer. You can't leave out health educators, personal trainers, and spa coordinators, along with chefs, nutritionists, and nurses. But as I enjoyed the sunshine while watering flowers, I discovered the unexpected health in landscapers.

I have a feeling that if you thought long and hard enough, you could find health in your profession. Now, some of the ones mentioned above are more obviously connected to healthcare. But many career paths would not necessarily be classified as health jobs, but they are. Take for example, landscapers.

Landscapers provide lots of obvious health benefits to our society: they color our world with flowers, trees, and potted plants, reminding us that among the ugliness that surrounds us, beauty can prevail. Landscapers plant our earth with oxygen-rich greens that purify our air and contribute to abundant health. And a beautiful landscape is a perfect cure to a not-so-healthy mood. But the unexpected health in a landscaper is that as we see health in a broader way, we can see that doctors can be dressed in more than scrubs. They can come without stethoscopes, M.D.'s attached to their name, and hospitals to call their work home. People who provide health don't need a fancy PhD.

My parents are landscapers. Neither one of them went to school directly for landscaping but both have been blessed with incredibly green thumbs (I think I might have a slight green tint to my phalanges now too, thanks to them!). Their backyard is an oasis in the middle of a city. It is serene, soothing, and in my opinion, one of the greatest doctor visits I could ever make an appointment for (actually, I am more of the walk-in type). I look around at the tranquility they created and I am reminded that not only is health realized in unexpected ways, but healthcare practitioners are sometimes unexpectedly clad as well.

We all have the gift of healing. We can create beauty and health for ourselves, our friends, our loved ones, even complete strangers. My parents are landscape doctors, some of my friends are teaching doctors, others are design doctors... Maybe I'm a writing doctor?!

So the next time you question your profession, your calling, or your contribution to this world, remember that you are a healer. You can help create and facilitate health in anything you work at. What really matters is not so much what you *do*, but how you are *being*.

In Memory of Health

Memorial Day is a day set aside to honor and remember those who fearlessly sacrificed their lives to protect our nation. My heart feels sad today for those families who have buried their sons, daughters, fathers, mothers, husbands, and wives. But I am reminded of the sometimes surreal, sometimes sad, but unexpected health, one discovers in memories.

Now, recalling times of great joy, blissful love, and world travel is obviously healthy: these make our hearts happy. Memories of good times elicit a positive experience throughout our beings. But not all memories bring us back to unimaginable happiness. In fact, some memories cause an overwhelming amount of sadness, anger, and grief. There are some recollections that at times, we would prefer to forget—or even to have never experienced. But the unexpected health in these less-than-ecstatic memories is that remembering our past is part of our healing... And being present to the healing in our lives is healthy.

Memorial Day is a day to remember—remember where we have been, what we have been through, and what we have learned in the process. We have memories so that we are able to navigate through the labyrinth that is our life.

Without memories, we are left with an empty hole in our hearts, a hole that is meant to house all of the memories our brains can hold on to. And even if these memories ended with an unexplainable, sad event, that is just one piece of the story.

I think about people I have lost in my life. I think about my grandmother and how I will never pass a berry bush without picking a berry, eating it, and then remembering how I used to pick these little fruits for hours, because I knew the more fruit I had, the better the pie she would bake! Yes, my grandmother died, and that is a sad memory. But my grandmother's story did not start, nor will it end, there. When I think of her, I do feel sadness. But I can contribute to the healthy inspiration she was in my life by allowing her legacy to live on through me. And the compilation of all of my memories of her are the only way I can keep her spirit alive. We never forget those whom we loved and lost. We're not meant to.

So the next time Memorial Day rolls around, remember. Remember those who are no longer with us. Be reminded of who they were while living in this world. Think about the healthy contributions they made in your life and the lives of others. And remember that you are who you are right now because of the people and experiences that have blessed your life so far.

A Knock-Down, Drag-Out Fight for Health

I am always up for a good old test of character. You know, those times of trials and tribulations that push every button we didn't even know we had? As often as I think I fail these tests, I am always game to get back out there and put my best foot forward in the character challenge. But one day, as I heard of squabbles between family and friends, I discovered the unexpected health in fighting while recalling a few of my own snarly times.

Sidenote: I am in no way referring to physical fighting or violence. There is nothing funny nor healthy about that. What I am talking about is that steam-coming-out-of-your-ears-from-irritation reaction to another.

For any of you who have ever fought (which is everyone!), you can probably list a few of its healthy benefits: fighting allows for honesty to shine through, even if the delivery is a little rough around the edges, a fight can create a completely different, healthier dynamic between two people, and a good old-fashioned fight infuses us with a much-needed perspective. But the unexpected health in fighting is that when we fight, we are being given a character test... And any test of our being is healthy.

Fighting brings up an array of emotions, past and present experiences, resentments, and any other feeling we have stuffed inside for way too long. That's why it becomes a fight. If we continuously discussed our frustrations and hurt along the way, a fight would probably never arise. But we are human. We silence ourselves when we feel we need to, even when we desperately want to shout our feelings. We take the quiet zone because we do not want to rock the boat. We choose to neglect our own feelings to preserve another's wants and desires. Most of us were programmed to be peacekeepers.

But sometimes, when life presents us with a last straw, we blow our lid, roll up our sleeves (figuratively, of course), and throw our verbal punches. Now of course, it is best to leave personal slander and low blows out of the fight, but once in a while, we need to let our truth be known, in whatever form we can relay it! We can only tolerate so much, right?! There comes a point in our lives when we must speak up, for the sake of our health. And when we speak up, we are not only freeing ourselves from stored negative energy, we are telling another (even in the form of a yell) that we love them so much that we will not tolerate behavior that causes us to love them any less.

So the next time you get into a fight, don't be too hard on yourself. Remember that when we fight with our loved ones, no matter what the topic, we are quarreling, not because of the hate we feel toward them, but because of the love we have for them. We love our loved ones so much that when hurt happens, we get mad. But at the root of our anger is the deeper meaning: we love. When we love, we get hurt. When we get hurt, we fight. So fight it out, that's okay... But then get back to the love.

So You Think You Can Heal?

It's funny what makes a person cry. Those who know me know I have a hard time shedding a tear or two. But then, with the most unexpected of circumstances, I can sob like a baby.

At times, I think the trigger is my mood or emotional sensitivity. Other times, I am moved by something I see, something I hear, read, or experience. While I sat and cried through portions of my favorite talent TV show, I discovered the moving, unexpected health in dancing.

Just to set the record straight, I am a *huge* fan of *So You Think You Can Dance*. I have never been touched by the compilation of choreography, music, and moves as much as I have when watching a routine on this show. Now of course, there are lots of obvious health benefits to dancing. Being able to dance is a great way to enjoy a healthy dose of physical movement. Dancing offers an outlet for kids and adults who prefer tap shoes to cleats, and dance creates an intimate connection between partners. But the unexpected health in dancing is that when the moves and the music touch a dancer, a story unfolds... And being moved (at times, to tears) by the stories of others is healthy.

We have so many outlets for expression in our culture, for storytelling. Of course, we often watch movies, read books, or see musical theater when we want to be told a story. But how often do you watch a lyrical jazz or contemporary routine and have to reach for the tissue box? Before *So You Think You Can Dance*, I would have said, "Never." But one of the few healthy aspects of these talent shows (and TV altogether) is that we are introduced to less-than-mainstream forms of emotional expression. This is because we can touch and be touched by so many art forms.

In fact, these forms of creative storytelling force us to pay attention. Of course, we could say that we are inundated with technology and media, and that's true. But we also experience overwhelming accessibility to be present to the stories that happen around us on a daily, an hourly, basis.

So the next time you see a preview for *So You Think You Can Dance*, consider that block of time a productive, healthy way to unwind. I receive no endorsements for my praise of this show, but I always receive a gift when I watch it.

Color Full

I have never easily conformed to your average business attire... I guess that is why I don't have a *typical* career. I have worked at jobs where I was required to wear a suit every day. You can imagine how well that went over after a while. Now that I am versed in the salon world, I see a similar dress attire: black. Wearing black in the salon industry makes a ton of sense. Black is a very forgiving color, so when you splatter color on your clothes, nobody notices. Black is also very chic, so you can pull off an edgier, more glam look (especially with the right accessories). But one day, as I waltzed around in anything but black, I discovered the unexpected health in color!

I have talked before about color, but have only referred to the shades of *wow!* on a wall. And as stated previously, color has an array of healthy qualities: being colorful brightens any room, no matter how dark and dreary; color shows off a beautiful eye color, hair color, and skin tone; and certain colors are associated with very healthy, very specific life meanings (a little book on feng shui would be really handy to have). But the unexpected health in color is that a color contrast, no matter how subtle or extreme, expands the lens through which we see the world. And seeing our lives with a rainbow of colors is healthy.

I wore a bright red shirt that day. Now, first of all, I never wear red. I don't know why I choose to limit my closet from including this vibrant, very cheerful color, but I do. Well, evidently on that day, I was in a red mood. I didn't feel particularly red, but apparently, it felt me. For some reason, I received compliment after compliment in this colored shirt. At the end of the day, I sat and thought about what drew people to *that* shirt, *that* color. I realized that my shirt elicited a happy feeling in others, a sense of brightness and being alive. My red shirt may have been a contrast to their otherwise blah, kind of grey day.

We all have days when life looks a little bleak, when we walk out of the house with our zipper down, when we arrive fifteen minutes late to every appointment no matter how hard we try, when we make one mistake after another. When these days come about, we need a little light to shine in our direction, a little color to brighten our perspective.

So the next time you wake up on the wrong side of the bed, consider perusing your closest for the brightest, most vibrant colored shirt you've got and wearing it! You just never know how a simple color in your shirt can be the best pick-me-up of your day.

On the Edge of
Our Seats of Health

I like to live on the edge of comfort. I prefer to have multiple activities, projects, and to-do's rather than be bored from a lack of happenings. Sometimes this requires a bit of multi-tasking, sometimes a bit of busyness, and at times, a bit of stress. But aside from some of the less-than-healthy aspects of living outside of my comfort zone, having my edges pushed is filled with unexpected health. I discovered the unexpected health in anticipation.

I thrive when movement is taking place. I very intentionally use the word "movement," instead of "chaos," because I *chose* all of these activities and events I am engaged in... And making the choice to participate in healthy experiences is healthy.

Anticipation gives us hope. The excitement that anticipation elicits creates enthusiasm for life. When we feel stuck in the mundane, we have the opportunity to anticipate what sort of health opportunities are just around the corner. Waiting in anticipation can be frightening; the unknown can cause anything from anxiousness to heart palpitations. But often, anticipation comes when we are waiting to see how a choice we made will unfold, allowing us to be witness to the unfurling of our life's plans.

Chaos is very different from anticipation. Chaos is like a tornado, making the world seem as if it is spinning wildly out of control right in front of your eyes... Not so healthy! But anticipation is that butterflies-in-your-stomach sort of feeling or like the wild-and-free feeling right before you bungee jump or skydive. It is that quiet faith that everything is as it should be but has not yet taken form.

So the next time you feel a little anticipation, be grateful. Know that you are pushing the edges of your comfortable life so that you can live to your fullest potential, your most expansive self. Make it a goal to feel a little anticipation every once in a while—or even better, every day!

Calendar of Clarity

I have discussed the many health benefits of Fridays. I have attempted to shift our perspective to focus on the healthiness of Mondays. But you know, on that day that many feel down, I find there is a plethora of unexpected health in Sundays.

Now some might say that Sundays can elicit a melancholy type of feeling. Many claim to get the Sunday blues because of the inevitable placement of this day. Even though Sunday is considered a day of rest, Sundays tend to be dedicated to the laundry, grocery shopping, and all other errands. But the unexpected health of Sundays is that this day, unlike any other, provides adventures... And having unchartered territories at your fingertips is healthy.

Sundays are a perfect excuse to explore your area and beyond. They even name car rides after Sundays—you know, a Sunday drive?! These days can be so much more than the last day of your weekend and they can be so much more exciting than a typical to-do-list kind of day. Sundays give us a reason to get in our cars and see the world, even if it's just a new neighborhood. Think about all of the activities you could do on any given Sunday: many go to church, you can take a drive, you can go away for a day trip, you can check out open houses (a fantastic way to get renovation ideas for your own digs), you can even pick a place you've never been to and go!

We have all been guilty of dreading the last day of our weekends. But while we spend unnecessary time and energy thinking about the finality of our weekend and the looming start to our work week, we are missing out on the precious expansiveness of time. Instead of focusing on what is about to end (our weekend), what would happen if we focused on what's in store for us?!

So the next time you wake up on Sunday with the disappointment that your weekend is almost over, remember that Sunday really is Funday. It doesn't have to be the ending of anything... Let it be the beginning.

Pedaling Toward Health

I bought a road bike quite a few years ago. I thought that bike riding was going to be my newest hobby. Although I love to ride my bike, getting me on the darn thing is another story. So my poor bike does not get nearly enough use. But I recently ran across a photo of a painting I saw on a wall in Ireland that caught my attention. I discovered the unexpected health in bike riding.

I do not need to blab about the health benefits of cycling: you know, cardiovascular health, muscle-building, outdoor air, and the adventure! But riding a bike offers so much more than physical health. In fact, I might argue that the mental health benefits of cycling might outweigh the physical benefits. As I so profoundly learned from a side-alley wall in Belfast in Northern Ireland, the unexpected health in riding a bike is that it is actually a way of living... And allowing the mundane to unravel the marvel is healthy.

"Every turn of the wheel is a revolution." Those eight little words caught my eye as I walked down a nearly abandoned alley in Belfast. In fact, this area housed get-away exits for the Irish during the Troubles (the war between Catholics and Protestants). As my navigator friend and I walked through this war-burdened city, learning the history while still feeling the underlying current of the Troubles, I couldn't help but be blown away by this saying etched on a wall. Yes, to pedal a bike, you must turn the wheel. The full circle turn is a revolution, literally! But to turn the tides of our lives, our country, our world, we must also change our position; we must move in a forward direction.

I think about this saying often. I even blew up the photo, framed it and hung it in my office to look at every single day. I visualize what a simple pedal will do. With a single revolution, I can be in a completely different location. So the same goes for mental cycling. When we put our life gears in motion, we can cause a revolution, a revolution of body, of mind, of spirit, of heart. We are born as physical beings. This means that we were created to move—move our bodies, our minds, and our hearts. We can manipulate our muscles while, at the same time, inspiring our minds. So while my legs moved my body on the streets of Belfast, my eyes allowed me to see the expansive potential we all have when we churn up the waters to move our waterwheels—our lives.

So the next time you think about participating in a physical activity like bike riding, do it mindfully. Remember that even the simplest activity, one that you may have never done with awareness, can be the most powerful, the most visual reminder of where you are, where you are going, and who you are being. Be big!

Cardiovascular Health

I would never have considered myself a runner when I was young. In fact, I hated playing basketball *because* of all the running it required. I ran track in junior high but stuck with the short fifty- and hundred-yard dash. But a couple of years ago, I decided to change that story I had told myself that I wasn't and couldn't be a runner. I really wanted to be someone who could come home from work, put on her running shoes, and unwind with a run. Well today, as I returned from a post half-marathon run, I discovered the unexpected health in, you guessed it, running.

Now if you had asked me before any of my races, I would have been at a loss for *any* health benefits of running. But after the heat exhaustion subsides, I remember why running is so healthy for us (as long as your knees are up for the run). First, of course, running improves cardiovascular health. Second, running is also great for maintaining one's optimal body size (optimal for an individual, *not* what the media tells us!). And third, just like cycling, running is a great excuse for being outdoors. But the unexpected health in running is that no matter how far or fast you run, you always come back to your starting point... And knowing that you are not running *away* from life but are pacing *with* it is healthy.

You always hear the unhealthy correlations with running: you know, like being told that you are "running away from your problems." While I think we are all guilty of that from time to time, I found that today, I wasn't running to avoid anything at all.

Let me explain: I wanted to take a hike one day. But once I got out into the oxygen-rich, fresh air, I couldn't help but want to run! I never thought I would say that... I actually *wanted* to run! But here's what changed: my perspective, and ultimately, my health.

In the previous year or so, I had gotten back into running. But my reasons for running had less to do with recognition and all to do with health. For me, running was a challenge, but becoming a runner was achievable. Sometimes in life, we need to challenge ourselves. We need to set goals and work toward them. This cycle of setting goals and achieving them help solidify a bigger life goal: that of continually transforming. Running, for me, is like breaking out of the chrysalis (the story) and realizing the butterfly that is waiting to unfurl its wings and fly.

Life is movement. We constantly change the scenery, adapt our environment, and set the pace for our next adventure. What we think we can achieve, we can!

So the next time you feel the desire to set a goal, like running, remember that what you think is unreachable may very well be right at your fingertips—or in your next pair of running shoes.

Nine Healthy Lives

I have another shout-out to my four-legged friends. Now, I have talked at great length about my dog. But I have a secret to confess: I am not just a dog person. I am also a cat person. So, I have discovered the unexpected health of cats.

For well over a decade, I had two little feline friends, one black and one white. I rescued these little feline friends when they were merely four and five weeks old. In case you were wondering, I never wanted two cats. When my little cat buddy Jordan died, I knew that I needed a very special cat to even come close to the cog (not quite cat, not quite dog, I called him cog) I had. When I buried him, I swore I wanted a cat that looked nothing like him... So I set out to search for an all-white cat (Jordan was black). When I found Riley, he fit into the palm of my hand. In fact, he fell asleep there. Of course, his little nap gave me plenty of time to decide I wanted him. But he came with a catch: because he was so timid, he could only be adopted with a friend. Looking back, I think that was the pet store's way of getting its customers to adopt more kitties that day, but whatever! So, I perused the cages, looking for a companion for the little white ball of fur resting in the cup of my hand. And there, peering out with her nearly crossed eyes was a little black and white furball with long white whiskers. "I'll take that one too," I said. And off I went with not one, but two kitty cats.

You might be wondering at this point what my cat story has to do with health. I have already discussed the health benefits of animals, so I will not regurgitate that information again. But the unexpected health in cats is that their individual, sometimes aloof, and oftentimes quirky personalities are a brilliant reminder of the balance we need in our lives... And being reminded to stay balanced is healthy.

As I have mentioned, my cats are very different from one another. One is adventurous, fearless, and stubborn. The other one is timid, cautious, and needy. But the two create a perfect balance. What I thought I could *never* replace in the *one* cat I had, I found in two. And isn't this lesson a fantastically healthy reminder for life? How many times have we put all of our eggs in one basket? How many people have been our all-in-all, our everything, only to come tumbling off that pedestal they should have never been on in the first place. We can put all of our hope into one thing, one job, one relationship, one period of time, one accomplishment. But this one event, person, or experience will not keep the seesaw that is our life in balance. We need the experiences of many, the lessons learned from multiple people, and the ups and downs of possibly numerous jobs to find our homeostasis, our balance, our resting place.

I used to question why I had two cats. I complain about the fur, the litter box, and the pillow-sharing. But then I stop and think about how grateful I am for the lessons they have taught me. I am amazed by the education and the health I have received from my four-legged friends.

So the next time you wonder why in the world you have your animal, remember that our feline and canine companions may be unable to speak, but the health they share and the balance they display need no words. All that is required are open eyes to be witness to the lessons.

Nodding Yes to Health

I have a tendency to be a yes girl. I have said this before. I can easily overextend myself, overbook myself, and be overly tired from all the commitments at the end of the day. But as I somehow manage to juggle way too many tasks, I discovered the unexpected health in being a people pleaser.

Being a people pleaser can be a daunting chore. It can take a toll on our health, our vitality, and our energy for life. In other words, being a people pleaser can be quite unhealthy. When we constantly try to please others, resentment and anger can build up inside. We can neglect our own wants and desires, devalue our time, and put ourselves on the back burner. But as unhealthy as being a people pleaser sounds, being a yes person is unexpectedly healthy because the more we say yes to life, the more opportunities we are presented with. And having endless opportunity and potential is healthy!

Let me clarify: I am in no way suggesting that we throw self-care to the wind and be at everyone's beck and call. But sometimes, when we agree to be inconvenienced, to put a little extra time or TLC into something that we may not want to do, we are creating an expansive receptivity to all that life has to offer.

Recently, I agreed to be a part of an event that was not exactly what I wanted to be doing, but I did so because I wanted to be the best possible supporter that I could. As I chatted it up with various individuals, I realized that my minimal inconvenience was literally throwing opportunities into my lap. All because I was trying to please others.

It is so easy to get wrapped up in our own world, in our own to-do lists, and our own needs. And don't get me wrong, there is great health in self-care. But sometimes, we need to practice a little care-for-others! I'm not suggesting we become a complete co-dependent society, but I do think we can tip the scales a little more toward community collaboration instead of individual achievement.

So the next time you have the opportunity (and I do mean opportunity!) to help out, to please another, do it! Give someone the gift of your time, your support, your love. Remember, the pay-it-forward system is the best banking system we've got!

Sugar-Coated Health

I could potentially call myself a nutrition expert. I have been formally educated about healthy eating and feel quite confident teaching others about vitamins and minerals, macro- and micronutrients, etc. If you were to ask me for nutrition advice, I would immediately suggest drinking plenty of water, eliminating sodas, cutting down on breads, pastas, chips, and any other white-flour substances, and would definitely recommend removing sugar from your diet as much as possible. But today, after a beautiful walk in the open air, I discovered the unexpected health in snow cones!

Well, let me explain snow cones: I'm not talking about your do-it-yourself Snoopy snow cone machine that we kids had growing up. (Did I just age myself?) What I am referring to is Hawaiian Shaved Ice...that fifty-plus flavored sugar syrup drizzled over shaved ice. If you have ever been to the fair, you've seen these little bits of icy heaven. You can get any flavor imaginable: from blueberry to bubble gum to tiger's blood (not sure what that would taste like!), there is a flavor for every palette. My favorite is a combo of blue bubble gum and pink cotton candy! Now of course, there is *nothing* nutrient-rich about this concoction. In fact, I am quite sure this is a dentist's nightmare (and any nutritionist, for that matter). But the unexpected health in snow cones—Hawaiian Shaved Ice, to be exact—is that these kid-approved treats can remind us of our youth... And reminiscing about times before life's pressures forced us to grow up is healthy.

When my family and I lived out in the Capay Valley of northern California, a little blue snow shack (yes, literally a blue shack) served the most refreshing Hawaiian Shaved Ice during the hot summer months. As a treat, my mom would drive me into town to get a little summertime snow cone. I never lost my love for these little ice treats. When I moved to Chico, California, for college, I found a little frozen yogurt shop that carried the very same sugary snack. So of course, I can never make a trip to Chico without treating my taste buds to a little blast from the past.

Of course, our diets should not be filled with simple syrup and deep-fried fair food. But sometimes, we crave a certain food not because of its nutrients but more because of the memories it brings up. I have so many health-filled memories from my times living out in the country. I have countless healthy memories from my time living in Chico. Sometimes, I want to go back to those times, to remember and reminisce about life in those areas, as a kid or a college student.

So the next time you crave a little nutrient-lacking food, think about why your belly may want it. It's okay to splurge once in a while, especially when fond memories are involved.

Packin' in the Health

My friends and I (and my dog, of course) love to hike. Together we have gone on too many hikes to count over the years. But one hike sticks out as one I will never forget. We were in Bidwell Park in Chico, California, the second-largest city park in the country—a fantastic place. There are endless trailheads, a huge creek with countless swimming holes all named alphabetically by animal names (we swam at Bear Hole), beautiful trees, tons of wildlife, and of course, fresh air and endless natural beauty. As we walked single-file next to the creek trail, I thought about my life and, of course, my health. While I took in the beauty and serenity of that place, I discovered the unexpected health of hiking.

You don't have to be a health guru to know that hiking is healthy for anyone. There is nothing unexpected about that insight. But hiking has some hidden, some less-than-obvious, health aspects to consider.

Hiking, especially in a beautiful park like Bidwell, tends to be a long jaunt. When you want to explore the natural world, it is often a couple-hour excursion. You pack your water, some snacks, a camera, and away you go. We were no exception. We wanted to hike to one of the most popular swimming holes, and even though it was ninety-plus degrees, we were on a mission to make the trek. We arrived at the well-known water hole, swam around, jumped off a few rocks, and then basked in the sun for a while before heading back to the car. On the way back, Lucca started favoring her paws. In fact, she was having trouble walking. This brings me to the unexpected health insight: hiking can sometimes put people (and animals) in risky situations, which leaves open an enormous door for humanity to reveal itself... And giving humanity center stage is healthy.

By midday, Lucca (being the medium-haired black dog that she is) was hot, tired, and paw-burned. I know my pup very well, and I could tell she was not feeling well—at all. I also knew we had quite a journey back to the car in the hot sun and on the hot ground. Now, I like to think of myself as rather strong, but there was no way I could carry my nearly forty-pound dog that far. Sensing my worry, one of my good friends swooped her up, threw her over his shoulders, and sweated his way—with her—back to the car. Imagine carrying a hairy, black, heavy, dirty dog, in the middle of the day, in the blazing sun, when it's not even your dog!

When we get ourselves (or our dogs) in a bind, it's amazing how the humanity of others can show up and unexpectedly support us. There was no way I could have helped my little furry friend today, but someone could. We do not always have to know all the answers or have the strength to fight our own battles; that's what friends, family, and loved ones are for. We are in each other's lives to be the wings when we need a little help soaring, or the arms when we need to be carried. We are not meant to live this life on our own. We will fail miserably and get lost on our lonely trailheads if we try.

So the next time you find yourself in a bit of a bind, pay attention to the helpers who show up to assist. Do not doubt if and when help will come. It will! We just have to be willing to let others help carry our loads—or our dogs.

Discovering Health Overnight

Remember when you used to wait for letters to come anxiously? I think back to my childhood and remember obsessively checking the mailbox if I knew a letter was on its way. The anticipation was nearly more than my impatient little self could stand! It was so fun to decorate letters, spray them with perfume (yes, I did that), and seal them with a lipstick kiss (did that too). I remember getting letters from my mom at summer camp, letters from boys I would meet at summer camp, and always letters from my best friend who lived far away from me (she was always much better at sending letters than I was). There was something so special, so individualized, about snail mail letters. But nowadays, we are crazy about email, instant messaging, and texting. In fact, I can't even remember the last time I sat down and wrote a letter (birthday cards don't count!). But one day, as I express-mailed a very important package, I discovered the unexpected health in FedEx.

After my nostalgic reminiscing about letters, you might wonder why overnight delivery services are so wildly healthy. Don't worry, I have asked myself that very same question. Speedy mail and package services like FedEx enable struggling procrastinators—not healthy. Companies like

Amazon, UPS, and FedEx feed this country's appetite for instant gratification. And with so many brown, yellow, and white delivery trucks trekking around this country, the air quality continues to worsen. But the unexpected health in the modern-day delivery service is that the faster we can send information, the quicker we can facilitate health and unveiling health ASAP is healthy.

I sent what I would call an "awakened" package through FedEx on that day. I also ordered a health supplement, and I received a picture of health from air mail a few days ago. All of these packages being sent and received are opportunities to share health, health information, health food, and health inspiration. I'm not saying that every package you ever send or receive is obviously healthy, but who knows what sort of joy or peace your delivery may be providing.

Receiving a letter is still a treat, don't get me wrong. But sometimes, we need to move the health process along. There are times when we need to put our health efforts into overnight mode, to kick health up to high gear. When we see an opportunity to put our health foot forward, we need to seize the moment and not a minute later.

So the next time you fret about the high costs of overnight, express, and three-day delivery, remember that you are paying a little extra to move health at the speed of life.

An Exfoliating
Mask of Health

Anger is a dead giveaway. There are no fooling feelings of anger. We may think we are tricksters when we burst out in fits of anger, assuming that our emotion is probably labeled when actually, it isn't. One day, as I took the roller coaster ride named P.O.'d (and I'm not talking about an address!), I discovered the unexpected health in anger.

I have already talked about the harm and the health of getting mad. But the emotion of anger is a little different. You see, getting mad helps propel us toward change. We become so uncomfortable with our annoyances that we are forced out of the comfort zones we may be lingering in. But anger is different. Anger can be more than unhealthy. In fact it can be downright toxic. Getting angry usually results in an eruption of irrational emotion, verbal vomit, and physical dis-ease (blood pressure rises, breath shortens, hormones get out of whack...). But surprisingly, anger has two powerful bits of unexpected health.

Let me explain: the first tidbit of health from getting angry is that when our body is storing anger, we have a physical sensation to release it. I found that I needed to let go of the anger I was holding inside today, so I made a crunch-away-your-frustrations salad for dinner—and of course, eating salad is healthy! Chewing is a known stress-reliever, so it is no coincidence that we may crave crunchy food when we are stressed or angry. This is one of our body's coping mechanisms for letting the anger out, while allowing nutrients in. Now, when we experience heightened senses (which happens when we are angry), our bodies have a harder time digesting food. But sometimes, we have to physically help our emotions along, even if we do not receive complete nutritional benefit. I experienced health today by both the nutrients I was receiving and the release I was witness to.

The second unexpected health tidbit from anger is that, as I mentioned above, anger is a dead giveaway. Anger is a mask for sadness, disappointment, and fear. And realizing the underlying messages of unhealthy behavior is healthy. If you think about what makes you angry long enough, you will undoubtedly discover that something deeper is triggering your "safer" feeling of anger. Oftentimes, getting angry is much easier than feeling sad, experiencing disappointment, and coming face-to-face with fear. When we get angry, we keep someone else at fault. We can divert attention away from ourselves and the root of our emotional upset. We keep the angry conversation at the surface instead of digging in deeper to investigate the cause of our anger trigger. When I sit with my anger long enough, what I find is that I am sad, disappointed, or scared. But for me, anger is a much easier emotion to access.

Anger is a complicated emotion that we all experience. What seems so obvious, like our anger, is actually wrapped up into a much tighter package of let downs, sad feelings, and fear-based thinking.

So the next time you get really angry, I have a couple of suggestions. First, when you are hungry, give your body physical release by snacking on something healthy and crunchy (although please don't eat *just because* you are pissed!). Second, have a conversation with yourself about what might be causing the anger outburst. For example, ask yourself what sadness, disappointment, or fear you may be feeling when something angers you. I think you may find that these two little health tricks may keep your body nutrient-rich and your mind richly nourished. If neither of those work, then let out a loud sound. Sometimes physically releasing anger through noise can work wonders.

Forget-Me-Not, Remind-Me-Always

As I have mentioned before, I live my life by my iPhone calendar. If I lost my phone, I would not know where to go, what time to be there, and I would have no clue what the heck it is I'm supposed to be doing.

It is rather sad that my days are directed by the *ding* reminders of my little electronic day planner. But today, as I had both virtual and physical taps of recollection on the shoulder, I discovered the unexpected health in reminders.

Now of course, reminders are healthy for obvious reasons, the most obvious being that they help us remember our schedules. This helps us stay on track, be on time, and remain focused. We experience health when we are able to respect our own time and the time of others. But the unexpected health in reminders is that tying that string around our finger of forgetfulness allows us to stay committed... And being committed to life is healthy.

I typically have many reminders throughout my day. Yes, one of the more in-my-face (and more annoying) ones was my iPhone calendar alerts. But every one of my *ding* reminders is also a commitment tracker of some sort. For example,

I had reminders about when to be at appointments. These reminders help me keep my commitment.

Non-electronically, I am also given physical reminders. I am constantly reminded about love, compassion, understanding, and acceptance. As much as I unconsciously avoid these reminders, I am faced with humanity's call to love on a daily, hourly basis. Most days, life does not allow me to avoid, judge, or separate myself from the humanness, the uniqueness, of all of us.

We are all unique clocks, and what makes us tick is completely individualized. I set my life toward a specific tick-tock pace, and that works for me. But I need reminders to direct my attention less on what people are doing or not doing, and more on how they are being or not being. This is the daily reminder I need set on my iPhone every day. Forget about the appointments, the to-do lists, and the dinner dates, if I cannot remember that we are all unique and that our journeys are not on the same path, then no calendar alert can direct me toward health.

So the next time you create a reminder, take the time to consider what you want reminding of in life. Yes, it is important to be reminded of your obligations, but it is even more vital (and even healthier) to be reminded of your commitment—your commitment to expansiveness for all. That is the best reminder, the greatest aspiration, we can ever dial into.

Outspoken Health Advocate

Okay, quick show of virtual hands: who likes speaking in front of a group? Getting up and gabbing in front of strangers (or even friends) is somewhat scary for many of us. But today, as I was forced to stand up and sell myself, I discovered the unexpected health in public speaking.

Now, public speaking can elicit quite a few unhealthy reactions. For starters, speaking in front of a crowd (or even a few people) can send someone into a state of serious panic—not healthy. Getting up and speaking in public can cause shortness of breath, excessive sweat, even blotchy skin—again, not healthy. There have been times that I was medically concerned about some of the speakers I have seen turn ghostly white from their fear of speaking in public. But the unexpected health in public speaking is that no matter how scared you may be to get up in front of a crowd, your words have the opportunity to create change. And having the courage to stand up and speak up for change is healthy.

Public speaking allows us to promote ourselves, our belief systems, our passions. When we have the opportunity to get up in front of a group, we are given undivided attention for which to relay whatever information, education, and inspiration we like.

We owe it to the health of our world to step out of our comfort zones, to stand up and speak up when necessary. If we are in the business of facilitating health, then we must be willing to walk through fear, to surpass mediocrity, and to open our mouths and educate, even if we are petrified to do so. I used to be fearful of public speaking. Now, I still get a little anxious, but I do it anyway because I know that what I have to say is important and could be life-enhancing.

So the next time you are given the forum to speak publicly, take it as an opportunity to share a little insight, a little education, a little health. When our intentions are clear and our hearts are in the right place, then we have nothing to fear. So stand up, speak up, and elevate awareness.

A Clean Bill of Health

Aah, Friday mornings. How great is it to wake up knowing that the weekend is upon us? I love the excitement that Friday mornings elicit. Every Friday morning I think: "What am I going to do this weekend? Am I going somewhere? Am I going to experience something great?"

For the most part, I try my best to plan a few fun (and definitely healthy) activities during any given weekend. But one Friday morning, as I arose, got dressed, went to work, logged onto my email, there they were, displayed in between my personal messages and work emails: unopened, unpaid... *bills.* As I calculated and paid all of my bills, I discovered the unexpected health in bills.

I imagine that bills are never the highlight of anyone's day. In fact, I bet that there are a large number of people who experience plenty of ill-health when bill due dates come around. But stuffed neatly in the self-addressed return envelope is the reminder that paying bills means that you are supplied with one of the very most basic needs in life, like food and shelter... And realizing the opportunities instead of the obligations we have in life is healthy.

As I snarled at the twenty-five various taxes, fees, usage charges, and whatever else these corporations want to tack onto my bills, I thought about how any service costs so much more because of all these hidden costs. But then I had an unexpected health insight: I can afford these hidden costs! Yes, it is incredibly annoying to pay an extra twenty dollars in fees I know nothing about, but what really matters is that I live in a country that even offers these luxuries that other countries know nothing about.

It is so easy for me to take for granted all of the health I am exposed to. I have a beautiful place to sleep, a reliable car to drive, family and friends who love and support me, and a career that is both fulfilling, financially stable, and pays the bills!

So the next time you open your plethora of bills, remember that although it may be irritating to pay for unknown fees, you are blessed to afford the service—and blessed with an address the bills get sent to.

An Ode to Dads

Dads are so unexpectedly healthy because their display of love is sometimes a little undercover. You don't always see their love coming through and sometimes you don't feel the impact until you realize what they've done. Moms tend to be more obvious displayers of love. My mom will grab my brother and I and lay a big kiss on our faces. She will celebrate our victories with parties and presents. And she will cry at any and every tear-jerking moment in our lives, or even a sentimental birthday card.

On the other hand, my dad is more of the quick, sometimes prickly kiss on the cheek kind of guy. He doesn't organize the parties and presents but is up at the crack of dawn preparing for the party, working hard after the festivities end, and providing the money to buy all the gifts. He may not cry at every heartfelt card he has ever received, but he is sentimental and supportive of all of our milestone moments.

Dads are like quiet hummingbirds (at least my dad is). You don't always experience their scattering of love until later, when you see the flowers of your life blossoming and blooming. Dads spread love, growth, and beauty just as moms do, but in a completely unique way, a man's way. My dad may not have made my lunches every day, but he made sure he was home for dinner every night.

Parents take such criticism—and they take it gracefully. Some get in trouble if they feed their baby the wrong way. Or if they work too much. Or if they are too tough. For me, the beauty and health in growing in, has been recognizing and realizing that my parents show their love in quite unique ways, but one is not stronger than another. During my teenage and early college years, I might have ranted and raved that my dad did not understand me. But what I have come to realize is that it was not him who didn't know me... it I who did not understand him. Life is so much sweeter when we can see. I *see* my dad—and I am grateful.

So the next time you think your parents are annoying, that they don't understand you or that they are totally old school, take a step back and widen your gaze. What you might be assuming about them may actually be your misunderstanding of them. They love you...even if they have differing ways of showing it.

Berry Healthy

Did you know there is less-than-obvious, unexpected health in berry vines? I'm not talking about the antioxidant-rich fruit that hangs on their prickly little fruit vines. That's obviously healthy. I'm referring to the actual vines themselves.

I have not come into combat (and I do mean combat!) with berry bushes since the last time I was in Oregon... And the last time I was in Oregon was to bury my grandma. But sometimes, the most beautiful, the most healthy, experiences we have are not free of hurt. The sting of sadness can prick our hearts just like a berry vine, but often, even in pain, there is health. Finding the health in hurt is healthy.

I always remember my grandma Lucille on her birthday. On her last one, she would have been a hundred and four years old. She died at the young-at-heart age of a hundred and although her body had decided it was time to rest for eternity, she was as strong-hearted on her hundredth birthday as I remembered her my entire life. Memories of my grandma blew through me often on her last day. I don't know if it was the combination of her birthday falling on the summer solstice or whether it was just a day of dedication to her life here on Earth, but I found myself reminiscing about my time with her.

My grandma made the best homemade berry pies and cobblers. And what made her pies and desserts so delicious (and healthy, I might add) was that the fruit came from the vines that our hands were stained purple and pink from picking. I remember picking berry after berry, trying to fill up a basket full enough to make a pie (it always took me longer because I usually ate half of my pickings). What a joy to see our hard work and berry vine battle scars pay off with a warm, crisp pie, fresh out of the oven.

My grandma's death was sad. She was the type of grandma people write stories about. You know, the one who knitted dolls (and made my dolls and I matching clothes), read stories, and taught real-life lessons about life, love, and fairness. She never missed a birthday, never forgot a special occasion, and never became frustrated while trying to teach my brother and I how to fish. I think the harshest word she ever said was, "Oh fiddles!" Some might choose another F-word for that statement, but not my grandma. She was as pure as the Oil of Olay she lathered on her skin.

After both of my grandmas died (fourteen hours apart from each other), I used their lives and their deaths as the canvas on which to write my application essay to my graduate program. They inspired me to apply to the program that I have since graduated from, which has completely changed my life for the better.

Life does not come without the thorns, the berry bushes. We are never guaranteed a life free of hurt, sadness, or disappointment. I am sad that my grandma will never meet her great grandchildren on this Earth. I am disappointed that she did not get to see how her granddaughter turned out. But I am thankful for the twenty-seven years I had with her. I am thankful for the berry vines. I would never take back the times I shared with her, picking berries near the river.

I am the woman I am, seeing life through the lens of love, because of her contribution to my life.

So the next time you get tangled in your own painful berry vine of sorts, remember that the hurt is only part of the story. There is so much health to experience in this lifetime. We just have to focus on the fruits of our journey.

Enhancing our Middles

Middles get a lot of attention. Let's see, there are like a hundred different belly-fat-burning supplements, exercise DVDs, and tummy-slimming clothing to help get rid of our unwanted middle sections. Middle children have been the topic of childhood development research. There have even been questions about the middle of sweets (like, what the heck *is* in the center of an Oreo?). But one day, as I looked at the calendar and realized that we were right in the middle of the year, I discovered the unexpected health wedged... in the middle.

There are loads of healthy opportunities at the beginning and at the end of any given year. We have New Year's resolutions to plan, start, and then *usually* fail by February (hey, I've worked in the fitness industry, it's true!). At the end of the year, most of us enjoy holiday time with family, friends, and time off from work. But the middle of the year is another time of year to experience abundant health... And realizing you can create health at any time on your calendar is healthy.

We shouldn't need a holiday or a time of year to practice healthy behavior. We can set goals and achieve monumental milestones on any day, during any month. In fact, the middle of the year is a perfect time for a little health. Why not make some mid-year resolutions? Without the hype and pressure of starting the year with a laundry list of to-do's, must-do's, and need-to-lose requirements, the middle of the year allows us to be mindful of areas we want to expand in our lives, without Oprah telling us to do so. Nobody is going to ask you what your mid-year resolutions are going to be because most are still stuck on the fact that they fell off the wagon of their own New Year's goals.

There are always going to be times when we feel like failures. It is unrealistic to expect that there will never be areas in our lives where we feel we could have done better, worked harder, and fought longer. But let's keep failure out of health goals. I believe that we cannot fail at health. We may make less-than-healthy choices in our lives, but that does not mean that we are failures or even that our health is failing. However, goals like New Year's resolutions do not come free of hype and unrealistic expectations.

So the next time you fail your New Year's resolutions, forget about them. Try setting some goals right now, even if it's right smack in the middle of the year. We need to create *more* opportunities for experiencing health, no matter what time of year it is. As we try and tighten up our physical middles, let's loosen up on our rigidity of time when setting health goals. Let's meet in the middle.

Give Health Some Credit

I love to travel. I might even say I was born with a wild curiosity for adventure. I love exploring new places, seeing new sights, and taking in unfamiliar scenery. I live for that stuff! It expands my mind and my heart, giving me a larger lens through which to see the world and a greater capacity to experience the bigger picture. But traveling requires money. Now of course, you can spend thousands of dollars on an elaborate trip or can skimp by on campsites and packed food, but either way, you must have a little green in order to leave your zip code. So today, as I thought about my future adventures, I discovered the unexpected health in credit cards.

Now hold on just a second! I am in *no* way suggesting that credit card debt is the way to go. In fact, there is quite a dis-ease of overspending and excess that has become an epidemic in this country. There is absolutely no health in living beyond your means, spending more than you have, or living a life on plastic. But the unexpected health in credit cards is that these credit card companies have endless spending perks. So if you are going to have a plastic card, at least benefit from the offers... And taking lemons to make lemonade out of any situation is healthy.

Let me explain: most of us have credit cards. We all don't live off of credit and we definitely don't all live beyond our means... But we all have at least one MasterCard, Visa, American Express or Discover card that takes residence in our wallets. These companies have helped get us Americans in a lot of trouble with no-interest charges, high spending limits, and easy pay-as-you-go plans... You pay what you can, and your total amount goes way up because of interest rates. But we could also thank these credit card corporations as well. They have given us at least a little payback for our spending. It's called... miles!

Credit card miles are fantastic! And to me, anything fantastic *has* to be healthy! I once looked over my upcoming travel plans, and two of my plane trips were paid with miles. Yes, I had to spend money to rack up these miles, but I would have spent the money anyway. Now, because of my Chase mileage account, I am flying high in the friendly skies for zero dollars.

It would be difficult to cut our credit cards and pay our way through life in cash, although Dave Ramsey would disagree. Sometimes we just need a little wiggle room with our money distribution. So credit cards, as harmful as they can be, offer a wonderful way to both spend as needed and save as wanted. As we spend, we save. As I had spent money the previous year and that year, I had been saving my miles. When I had travel plans coming up, I could go away without breaking the bank.

So the next time you pull out your credit card, make sure you are getting some return on your investment. If you don't have a credit card with some sort of payback plan (miles, dividends, cash, whatever), get on the internet, research the best give-back program out there, and transfer your card! In tough economic times, if you will spend money, at least have your money working for you.

Writing Our Own Health Ticket

Do you ever end a perfectly good lunch or dinner date with a little white piece of paper flapping on your windshield? I have. And it was at that moment (okay, maybe more like five minutes later... I needed the first four minutes to whine) that I discovered the unexpected health in parking tickets.

Yep, we can actually come to appreciate that little piece of slick paper. Seriously, after double-checking to make sure the parking people had the right time, some why-me lamentations, and some choice curse words offered to those obsessively punctual meter maids, I have found that a bit of health can be experienced with tickets, unexpectedly. You see, although being the recipient of a ticket can be full of unhealthy feelings, the unexpected health in a parking ticket is that tickets force us to contribute to communities. And being a part of a community by any means possible is healthy.

Did I want to contribute forty dollars to the city? Not necessarily. In fact, I could have thought of a million other ways I would have liked to have spent that money. But do I want cities to thrive, to continue growing, expanding, and providing more opportunities for its dwellers and beyond? Absolutely!

Life has a funny way of allowing us to give back sometimes. Sometimes we give back by feeding someone else's meter, so they don't get a ticket. Other times, we give back by force, say, with parking tickets. But no matter how we give back to our communities, we will undoubtedly experience health.

So the next time you are forced to give back, try considering the gift you may be contributing. Yes, a lunch that extended for two minutes longer than planned might have cost you a ticket, but I am willing to bet that more often than not, the conversation and the connection are worth the money... And then some!

Sweat Your Health

My body typically runs a little cool. What that translates to is a never-ending struggle for a comfortable temperature in the car for both me and my passenger, the need to always bring a sweater (which I rarely do!), and a must-pack item in the winter: slippers. But in the summertime, I have the opposite problem and therefore discovered the unexpected health in sweating!

It is interesting how body temperatures can fluctuate so dramatically. When it is cold, I am particularly cold. When it is hot, I sweat like that person in your cardio bootcamp class who flips their sweat all over the class. But sweating has all sorts of health benefits: working up a good sweat means we are doing some sort of activity; sweating eliminates toxins through our skin, maintaining the healthiest inner landscape of our bodies; and having sweat beads trickle down our faces means that our bodies can return to homeostasis healthfully. But the unexpected health in sweating is that when you are dripping with that salty liquid, you are participating in life. And being reminded of your existence and participation on this planet is healthy.

As much as I feel like a dirty mess when I am sweating, there is this gratifying feeling of happiness, of health, that I experience. Being able to sweat means I am able to physically move my body, a luxury that not everyone has. I can work hard and play hard, and having that opportunity allows me to contribute my gifts, my ability to work, even my sweat, for a greater purpose.

So the next time you get annoyed from sweating bullets, remember what a gift it is for those of us who are lucky enough to have full use of our bodies and minds! So share your talents, give away the gift of a little time, even if it includes a heavy dose of sweat.

Meeting Health in the Middle

Do you ever have days when you look at the clock and wonder where the time went? I imagine that all of us have experienced this kind of day at some point in our lives. My days are often filled with various commitments, obligations, and opportunities, and in one of those days, I discovered the unexpected health in meetings.

Meetings can be associated with some ill feelings. Meetings tend to be long and can feel like a waste of time when participants stay too long on one subject. Meetings can be a reenactment of the school days' bullying system of getting one's way. And a meeting can be so focused on the protocol that quality, inspiration, and innovation can be lost. But the unexpected health in a face-to-face are that meetings provide an outlet for sharing at a more intimate level... And having a forum for life enhancement is healthy.

We have this amazing opportunity to create platforms for health conversations in just about anything we do. It is not necessary to be in the narrowly defined health field in order to have meaningful meetings. As I have stated before, we are all in the health business because we are all human beings living and thriving (or trying to) on this planet. And the more we realize the health business we are in, the greater the opportunity we have to infuse health into everything we are a part of.

So the next time you head to another meeting, think about how health can be added to the agenda. Because in years to come, it will not matter what the quarterly budget was, what the employee handbook says, or what the monthly special will be... The only meetings that will matter in the future are those we have with ourselves *now*. These are the meetings that ask us the questions about how we are living and loving in this world. The extent to which we do these things well is the depth of health we can and will experience. So make your meetings matter!

Health's Number-One Fan

There is something surreal and healthy about professional ball games. They always seem to bring me back to my younger years. I loved the sounds of the screaming fans, the noise the ball made when it hit the bat, even the vendors yelling out their featured goods for sale. "Peanuts, get your peanuts!" I loved that! And yes, there is unexpected health in being a sports fan. Because seeing the passion, commitment, and dedication shared by the thousands (and tens of thousands) is healthy.

Sports fans are a passionate bunch. Dedicated World Cup watchers wake up at 5 a.m. to see a game. Diehard football fans will paint their faces, bodies, and cars to show their allegiance to a team. And rambunctious hockey fans will bang their hands against the plexiglass when the opposition is in their space.

It's amazing to watch people so passionately dedicated to a cause. I love to see grown adults get as excited as kids when something, someone, or some event ignites a wild enthusiasm inside them. Wouldn't it be great if this uninhibited appreciation of sports was as popular, as appreciated, as striving to live our life's greatest purpose? How great would it be if people stood up for their health and that of the world around them with the enthusiasm of those doing the wave at a baseball game?

It's easy to throw passion into sports, to be so heavily invested in the betterment of a sports team, to be overly concerned with player injuries, to talk *ad nauseam* about the livelihoods of professional athletes. But why does it seem so hard to be concerned about our own health? Why do we default to talking about the health and the lives of total strangers like pro athletes instead of having those self-health conversations?

Of course, there is nothing wrong with being a sports enthusiast. In fact, I happen to think having passion, no matter what the cause, is healthy. I would love to see that passion, commitment, and dedication that we pour into our sports teams trickle down toward our own playing field. The game of life is happening every moment, and I don't know about you, but I want Row 1, Section 1 seats for it.

So the next time you feel your enthusiasm for your favorite sports team come to you, try to use the same enthusiasm for the Game of Health!

Health to No End

As you can imagine, sometimes it's easy to find health in unexpected ways. Other times, when a day or week is full of activities, weekend travel, and life, trying to find the miracle in the mundane can be a little more difficult. In fact, there were times when I just downright didn't want to type any sort of anecdote about health or life. But as the finality of this project approached, I was overly aware of the unexpected health in endings.

Endings are not always associated with Disney's version of happy-ever-after. We do not always experience ecstatic joy when something ends—a relationship, a home, or a career. In fact, there is a lot of sadness that can be associated with endings. Think about the last day of a long-anticipated vacation. When that happens to me, I know I am not leaping for joy when packing my bags to return home to responsibility and requirements. But there is unexpected health in endings because there is actually no ending to anything in life... And realizing that every ending is merely a pause before the start of something new is encouraging—and healthy!

Life is not a compilation of periods at the end of a sentence. Instead, it is a book of colons, semicolons, dashes, and exclamation points! Whenever something ends, we are given a clean slate, an opportunity to start a whole new journey. When finality arrives, we should prepare ourselves because something else is coming soon, something to build on our previous experiences, our past relationships, and our most recently finished work.

When we do not hold on so tightly to our fear of the unknown, endings suddenly become less scary. We start to see the connections between the start of one thing and the completion of another. Life truly is cyclical.

So the next time you feel an ending drawing near, remember that what may be finished from one vantage point could be the beginning of a whole new adventure.

Sibling Satiety

sa·ti·e·ty (n): "The condition of being full or gratified beyond the point of satisfaction."

I can definitely relate to feeling full, like when I eat too much at my favorite restaurant. But how often do I feel satiated—"gratified beyond the point of satisfaction?" Recently, I did feel this overwhelming sense of abundance, and that happened when I discovered the unexpected health in brothers.

I find the sibling connection to be quite fascinating. My brother and I are not twins, although people used to think we were. We do not spend all our free time together, do not have the same interests, and do not always enjoy the same activities (he hunts animals while I seem to collect them). In fact, there were times in our lives when my mom probably said that we had all sorts of unhealthy encounters.

I always wanted to be around my brother from the time I was a little girl. I have always loved my big bro. I couldn't hang out with him enough. But unfortunately, he didn't seem to share the same sibling enthusiasm! As we have grown up, our connection has grown strong too. But the unexpected health in brothers—or siblings—is that they are our lifers for the good or the bad, and having someone (or someones) in your life for the long haul is healthy.

Siblings are also the only connections we have to our family once our parents are gone. No one knows the stories, the memories, and the life you lived except for your brother or sister. My brother and I can call each other and with just a few words of prompting, can recall the same memory, the same funny story, even the same location. No one else has that incredibly healthy ability to remember life like the person who has shared it with you since the day you or they were born.

My brother and I are different and that is okay. I may not agree with everything he does, and he absolutely does not agree with all that I do. But no matter what, we are connected for life. We cannot detach from our oneness as brother and sister. Even when we choose to embark on journeys, we are constantly sharing one story, the story of our lives as siblings.

So the next time you feel resentment for your siblings or wonder how on Earth you could be related, remember that the person who shares the same gene pool is a lifer. My brother has been with me since the day I was born and I am grateful for his presence in my life. He is one of the greatest health benefits I have ever experienced.

If the Shoe Fits, Keep the Box

I used to be a CBS. I'm not talking about being dedicated to specific TV networks (although *Beverly Hills 90210* used to air on CBS so maybe I am a diehard fan!). No, this acronym stands for something a little more detrimental to the wallet. I used to be a Compulsive Buyer of Shoes.

In high school, you could find every color of the rainbow decorating my closet floor. I had powder blue shoes, I had shoes covered in flowers, I had red shoes, black shoes, brown shoes, boots, flip flops, heels, flats, tennis shoes... My feet were never boring! My mom would cringe any time we would even approach a shoe store. And packing? How do you find a bag big enough to carry a weekend's worth of clothes and all the matching shoes? Let's just say I never had carry-on luggage.

I have thankfully grown out of my shoe fetish, partly because my feet get too tired and sore when I'm wearing three-inch heels and partly because I just can't fathom spending the money on shoes that aren't practical. But, as I was cleaning house, I found, packed away at the back of my closets, some refreshingly, nearly financially redeeming unexpected health in shoeboxes.

Shoeboxes are usually packed full of mementos, vignettes of specific times, events, and people in our lives… And heartfelt keepsakes promote health. I have had lots of shoeboxes in my life. I had a shoebox for every boyfriend, which was filled with cards, notes passed in class, poems… You know, the usual mushy stuff. I may still have one or two of those shoeboxes. But sometimes, shoeboxes were also beneficial because once the relationship ended, a shoebox fits neatly into a recycling bin (yes, sometimes the healthiest action you can take is to get rid of old keepsakes).

Recently, I found a shoebox full of somewhat unrelated yet profoundly meaningful times in my life: my college graduation tassel, my best friend's wedding invitation, an inspirational note from one of my past volleyball coaches, and my welcome letters to both my undergraduate and graduate colleges. I may never create a scrapbook to visually display all of these special times in my life, but I don't have to. I know that stacked in one of my rooms will be a bright orange Nike shoebox that will safely keep all of my memories (at least those I want to remember) in one location.

Health is a two-way street. Sometimes health means holding on to treasures—special people, special memories, and significant times that we never want to forget. Other times, the most health-filled act we can do is let go. Some people in our lives aren't meant to stay forever. Some memories and events we hold on to can keep us stuck, and the best propeller of change is to clean house of those memories to make room for new memories to be made. The trick is to learn to decipher which route is healthier to take—holding on or letting go.

So the next time you run into an old memento and you decide that those keepsake baseball cards, love letters, and invitations are worth saving, shoeboxes can be snug little keepers of those healthy times.

Epilogue

We have now reached the end of my journey to chronicle the gratitude, the health, and the happiness that life keeps delivering to us every day. But if you think I stopped looking for the good in my daily life, you'd be wrong. Once you get started on this journey, there is no turning back. Many years have passed now since I started this practice. And every day, I am reminded of how essential it is to see the good around me, in order to keep me going on this crazy journey we call life.

Many stories in this book unraveled the joy in everyday moments. Let's see: I lost my dog, I painted my office (and have now painted another one), I went on trips both in the sky and by car, I celebrated birthdays, anniversaries, and engagements with friends. I was humbled, I was a loser, I went out to eat, I got "high," I said no, I let go. I danced, I anticipated, I waited. I talked about my mom, my dad, my brother, my friends, and my "family," both here and in Heaven. I squawked on and on about my dog, I was moved by the metaphors of my cats. I was wrong, I was inspired, I was changed.

Many things have happened since then, all of which I am eternally grateful for. I embarked on this journey while I was in my early thirties. I had not yet met my husband and I had not yet become a mommy. I lived with roommates and my main responsibility was my dog and two cats. Life back then seemed a whole lot simpler. Even though many of the stories would have had different characters had I written this in current time, the moral to the story is still the same: happiness, joy, and health is ours for the taking. Our life's happiness—or misery—is about perspective. It's about finding the good in some of the goofiest places.

But the journey toward joy does not end here. In fact, it is only just beginning. My goal for you and for me is that we all change our eyewear, put on a new pair of lenses with which to see the world, and view our surroundings with a set of expansive eyes. More importantly, I wanted to share my vision of health, my view of well-being that is numberless, timeless, and at times, effortless. Sometimes, a perspective change is the healthiest metamorphosis we can go through. Oftentimes, it's all we've got to work with.

We should all continue searching for meaning in this lifetime. So whatever the reason may be for your searching, remember that this life goes by fast. We should not sit back and repeat the same negative patterns over and over again. It is time for a new perspective, a new vision of health, and a new story. Let's open our eyes to the health—the joy—that surrounds us.

Now it is time for you to find your own ways of seeing the health in your day-to-day life. Write it down and come back to it over and over and over again. You will not be disappointed, because once you get used to flexing that gratefulness muscle on the daily, it becomes hard to stop. We all learn to do things by repetition. When you first learned how to write, you had to focus so hard on spelling your name. But now you don't even have to think about it.

It's the same thing with gratefulness and health. Once we get used to doing it every day, it becomes second nature.

Of course, there will be days when our perspective will be foggy... And I anticipate those days indefinitely. But we can be acutely aware of the health we facilitate or negate for ourselves. We can consciously make the choices to create and sustain health in our lives... And we can be more awake to when we are not taking care of ourselves or caring for the people and the world around us. When you find yourself getting sad or frustrated as we all do sometimes, remember that your gratefulness muscles are sitting right there in your toolbox of life, ready to teach you lessons that will empower you to live life more intensely, more beautifully, more healthfully.

Eventually, you will surprise yourself by looking at things that once made you anxious, angry, or confused, and finding that they now make you excited, inspired, and awe-struck. And I will be waiting for you, eager to read about the many ways you have found unexpected health at the bottom of your purse, in the far corner of your desk drawer, and in the highest reaches of your sky.

Acknowledgements

To properly acknowledge and thank all of the incredible people who were a part of this book, I need to start at the beginning. Like, the very beginning. Mom and Dad, you have always been my biggest cheerleaders. Mom, you would have been like the flyer on those cheer squads. You know, the ones getting the most recognition because they are flipping and flailing about in the air? That's how you have been for me my whole life. You were the first to volunteer for all the field trips (dear Lord, you must be a saint). You were at every game, every ballet class and piano recital, every volleyball tournament, softball tournament, and every other thing I was a part of. Thank you for supporting me in everything, no matter how lame, how early, or how uncomfortable the seating might have been.

Dad, you have also always been my greatest cheerleader, but you were more of the base in the cheerleading squad. I'm actually not sure why I am using cheerleading metaphors because I have never been a cheerleader in my life. You're welcome for having one less sport to attend. Anyway, your cheerleading style was the more silent but constant type. You too never missed a game, a tournament, or a recital. You may not have chaperoned the field trips to the Capital, but you never wavered in your unending support of whatever sport or function I was a part of.

You both taught me early on that I could achieve just about anything I put my mind to. You encouraged me to dream big and instilled the confidence in me to go for it—whatever "it" might be. I honestly cannot thank you enough for giving me such an invaluable gift. The gift of confidence, of courage, of ability, and of humility, because lord knows I failed at plenty. But you taught me to get up, wipe the dust off my tutu, and try again.

There were plenty of teachers and coaches who encouraged the same determination and drive that my parents did, but I could not have written this book without the fire and passion for writing that was ignited by my college professor at California State University, Chico, Dr. Lyn Lepre. Lyn, I didn't even know that I wanted to be a writer before taking your first magazine writing course my junior year. But once I started typing, I never looked back. You told me that I was a great writer. You encouraged me to send my articles to big time magazines in New York and I did. You told me to write for the college newspaper and I did. All of these experiences gave me what I needed to start seeing writing as a real career path. You introduced me to a world that I love so much and you believed in me the entire way. Certain teachers and professors leave an impact on us that changes the trajectory of our lives forever. Lyn, you have always been that professor to me.

As you know, I wrote this book before I was married and before I had children. My stories consisted of adventures with my friends, outings with my niece, and lots of time with my dog. To all of you friends who recognize and remember the journeys from these pages, thank you! You were such an integral part of the lessons I learned from the times we spent together. For many of us, we have grown up together. Some of you I have known most of my life. The times we shared and the memories we made are ones I will never forget... And now that you have this book, you won't either!

But one friend cannot go unmentioned and that is my childhood friend Megan. Megs, you have known me almost my whole life. No really, we met when I was three years old and you were two and a half, so just remember who is older (and I always like to say wiser). You have always encouraged me to go after my dreams, whatever they were. You always had faith in my ability, even when I did not share that same faith (you thinking I have a good singing voice is still beyond me!). Whenever I shared a wild and crazy idea with you, you rarely, if ever, shot it down. You listened, you encouraged me, and often, you got right in there with me to see it to fruition. Thank you for dreaming big with me. Thank you for being the friend who encouraged me to open up my wings and fly.

To one of my greatest mentors, Kathy, who helped me discover who I am at my core. You were one of my very favorite people in the world and was another one of those cheerleaders whom I owe so much gratitude. You helped me see the world as it should be, not as it was. You opened my eyes to holistic health and nutrition, and let me just say I will never look at organic skincare the same. You left such an imprint on my life and your death at age fifty still makes me feel like a piece of me is gone. But I know we will meet again one day.

This book would not be what it is today without the dedication and diligence of my publicist Lyda Mclallen. From our first meeting, she just "got me." She understood me, what I was about, and what I was trying to say. Every suggestion, re-write, even font type, echoed my personality and writing style down to my overuse of punctuation and those cute little ellipses (oh how I love them... and side thoughts using parentheses). Thank you for believing in me and for pouring out your heart into this book. I can feel it, even though we are across the country from one another.

Lastly, I have to send some major shout outs, fist pumps, and mostly hugs, kisses, and snuggles to my family. To my husband, Damon, you never cease to amaze me. You have never, not for one second, tried to hold me back from dreaming big and going after life in a major way. You and I could not be a more perfect match. You have come alongside my parents in being my biggest cheerleader (although imagining you in those tight pants the guys have to wear makes me laugh out loud hysterically). You are the first to tell me to think bigger, expect greater, and accept nothing short of amazing. You celebrate with me in all my small victories and are understanding when I am typing away, reading, or researching at night when you are trying to sleep. You are game for anything I want to try (everything from being vegan to mindfulness classes to farm life) and you do it with enthusiasm (mostly) and positivity. I love you more today than ever.

To my birth children, Presley, Ryan and Joshua, you are the light of my life. I literally thank God every single day that He gave me you three. You are loving, kind, thoughtful, generous, and also hilarious in your own unique ways. I pray that I make God proud by raising you to be game changers, earth shakers, and to be the generation that finally gets this world turned right side up. You are all truly the light of the world and the salt of the earth. May you be the purveyors of this land today and always. I love you all with every ounce of my being.

To my step children, Kaden and Kendall, you have been two of my greatest teachers. You welcomed me into your life when you were just four and six years old. You are beautiful creations of God and are some of the kindest little (not so little anymore) humans I know. It couldn't have been easy to always share your dad with me and then twins and then one more. But you always surprise me with your love and dedication to our family. You have patience like saints and are game for every silly family night we have, every weird holiday tradition I insist we partake in, and every garage sale I drag our family to on Saturday mornings (you have to admit, you have gotten some pretty cool stuff... Well, not really). I have loved watching you grow into the incredible teenagers you are and know that God has amazing plans for both of your lives. I love you both so much and you make me so proud!

And one more lastly (I promise), I have to end this acknowledgement with a heartfelt RIP to my sweet, silly, and spastic pup, Lucca Jean. You were my faithful companion (think die-hard fan) for twelve years and you just might have taught me more about myself, life, and love during those years than anyone or anything else. You were one crazy girl, but dang, I loved you. And to my funny and furry Siamese cat, Riley, you too brought me so much joy, so many memories, and a lot of funny stories. Rest in peace my blue-eyed boy.

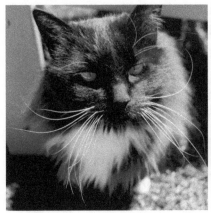

Bentley

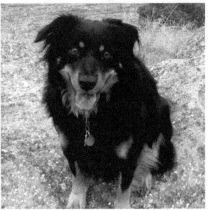

Lucca

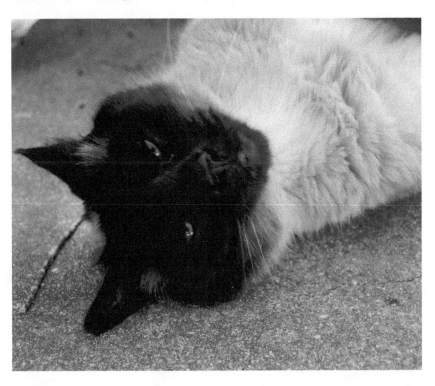

Riley

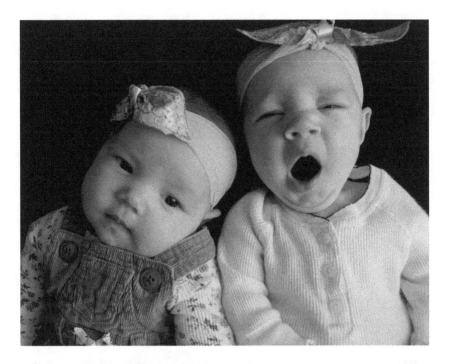

Ryan and Presley

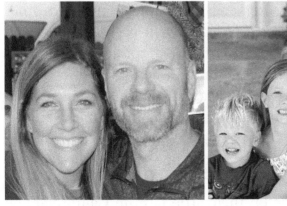

Damon and me

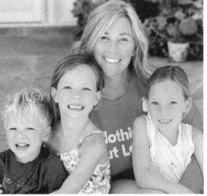

Joshua, Presley, Ryan and me

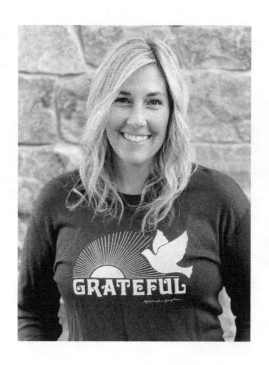

JAIME L. MATHEWS has been a writer for over twenty years. Her love of writing began while attending California State University, Chico. After college, Mathews pursued other business ventures but eventually went back to school and received a M.A. in holistic health education. But her love of writing never left her, so after a few years of a writing hiatus, she started writing again. This time, she launched and published a monthly healthy living magazine. Mathews eventually retired, as she was about to embark on her greatest adventure: parenthood. She is the proud parent of twin girls, a toddler boy, and two step kids. Mathews finds daily gratitude on their little farm in California. She and her husband soak up the sun while watching their children living life and spending time with all of their furry and feathered friends.